Pocket Reference to Early Rhe

Pocket Reference to Early Rheumatoid Arthritis

Paul Emery
arc Professor of Rheumatology
Academic Unit of Musculoskeletal Disease, University of Leeds,
Leeds Teaching Hospitals Trust, UK

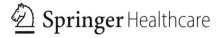

Published by Springer Healthcare, 236 Gray's Inn Road, London, WC1X 8HL, UK
www.springerhealthcare.com

British Library Cataloguing-in-Publication Data.

A catalogue record for this book is available from the British Library.

ISBN 978 1 85873 448 4

Although every effort has been made to ensure that drug doses and other information
are presented accurately in this publication, the ultimate responsibility rests with the
prescribing physician. Neither the publisher nor the authors can be held responsible
for errors or for any consequences arising from the use of the information contained
herein. Any product mentioned in this publication should be used in accordance with the
prescribing information prepared by the manufacturers. No claims or endorsements are
made for any drug or compound at present under clinical investigation.

Commissioning editor: Dinah Alam
Project editors: Hannah Cole and Alison Whitehouse
Designers: Joe Harvey and Taymoor Fouladi
Production: Marina Maher
Printed in Great Britain by Latimer Trend & Company Ltd.

Contents

Author biography

Paul Emery is Arthritis Research Campaign Professor of Rheumatology and Head of the Academic Unit of Musculoskeletal Medicine at the University of Leeds, as well as Clinical Director (Rheumatology) at the Leeds Teaching Hospitals Trust in the United Kingdom. He graduated in medicine from the University of Cambridge and completed specialist accreditation in internal medicine and rheumatology. He completed his thesis on the immunopathology of rheumatoid arthritis at Guy's Hospital, and then served as Head of Rheumatology at the Walter and Eliza Hall Institute in Melbourne. He was senior lecturer in rheumatology at the University of Birmingham, UK from 1987–1995 until his present appointment.

Professor Emery has served as a member of several education committees including the Senior Advisory Committees of the Royal College of Physicians, the MRCP Part 1 Board. He is currently the President of EULAR, a past member of the Scientific Committee and Chairs the MRI imaging group. He has served on the editorial boards of several journals, including *Rheumatology, Arthritis and Rheumatism, Annals of the Rheumatic Diseases, Clinical and Experimental Rheumatology, Clinical Rheumatology* and *Modern Rheumatology (Japanese Rheumatology Association Journal)*.

He is a recipient of the Roche Biennial Award of Clinical Rheumatology, the Rheumatology Hospital Doctor of the Year award 1999 and the EULAR prize 2002 for outstanding contribution to Rheumatology research. Professor Emery's research interests centre around the immunopathogenesis and immunotherapy of rheumatoid arthritis and connective tissue diseases. He has a special interest in the factors leading to persistent inflammation. He has published over 650 peer-reviewed articles in this area.

Chapter 1

Rheumatoid arthritis: an overview

Rheumatoid arthritis is a chronic systemic inflammatory arthritis of auto-immune origin that affects primarily the synovial joints, usually in a symmetrical pattern. It is the most common and most serious of the inflammatory arthritides, and it dominates clinical rheumatological practice (Silman 2002). Current evidence shows that prompt diagnosis and early instigation of definitive disease-modifying treatment can delay or avoid progression and enable patients to retain function that would otherwise be lost in this progressive and frequently disabling disease.

Incidence

Rheumatoid arthritis is estimated to affect between about 0.5 and 2% of the population worldwide (Alamanos and Drosos 2005, Emery 2006, Sommer et al. 2005).

Broadly speaking the disease is equally common worldwide, although there is some evidence of variation, with lower prevalence rates in southern Europe than in northern Europe and North America (Alamanos et al. 2006). There may also be lower rates in developing countries than in the developed world, a finding that has been attributed to environmental effects of urbanisation, although the precise causes are not known (Kalla and Tikly 2003). Some studies have reported a general trend for a decrease in frequency (Doran et al. 2002), more specifically in countries with high rates of disease (Alamanos et al. 2006) although such a trend is far from certain (Silman 2002). However, the small number of studies for most areas of the world and the lack of incidence studies for developing countries means that knowledge of the global epidemiology of rheumatoid arthritis is limited (Alamanos et al. 2006). UK data are summarised in Figure 1.1.

Rheumatoid arthritis in the UK

- 24 new cases of rheumatoid arthritis per 100,000 of the population per year [a]
- > 580,000 people have rheumatoid arthritis [b]
- Women 2–3 times more likely to be affected than men [c]

Figure 1.1 Rheumatoid arthritis in the UK. [a]Wiles et al.1999, [b] National Audit Office 2009, [c] Symmons et al. 1994.

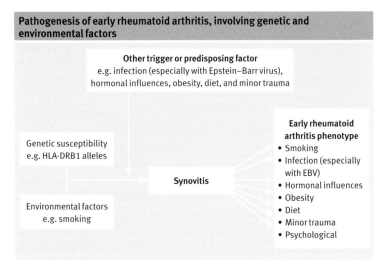

Figure 1.2 Pathogenesis of early rheumatoid arthritis, involving genetic and environmental factors. EBV, Epstein–Barr virus. Adapted from Pratt et al. 2009, with data from Pratt et al. 2009, Lee et al. 2007, Balandraud et al. 2004.

Aetiology and pathophysiology

The precise aetiology of rheumatoid arthritis is not known but it is complex and multifactorial, and involves both genetic and environmental components (Lee et al. 2007) (Figure 1.2).

Genetic factors

The disease is known to cluster in families, and those with a first-degree relation with rheumatoid arthritis are between two and 10 times more likely to have the disease than the general population (John et al. 1998). A genetic basis for this familial preponderance is confirmed by the observation that the concordance for rheumatoid arthritis in monozygotic twins is about 15%, up to five times the concordance in dizygotic twins (Pratt et al. 2009). Certain alleles at the human leukocyte antigen (HLA)-*DRB1* locus are known to be associated with susceptibility to rheumatoid arthritis and with the presence of autoantibodies, notably rheumatoid factor and antibodies against cyclic citrullinated peptide (anti-CCP antibodies or ACPA) (Gregersen et al. 1987). For example, *HLA-DRB1*401* and *DRB1*0404* are associated with radiographic erosions (Weyand et al. 1992).

Other genetic associations have also been identified (Pratt et al. 2009) (Figure 1.3). In Europeans, about 50% of genetic susceptibility to rheumatoid arthritis is contributed by two genes: *HLA-DRB1* and *PTPNN2* (Pratt et al. 2009).

Environmental factors

A number of environmental factors have been suggested as predisposing to or triggering rheumatoid arthritis (Figure 1.2). Of these, smoking is the only one that has been reproducibly linked to an increased risk (van der Helm-van Mil et al. 2007a) and only in patients with anti-CCP antibody (ACPA) positive disease (Klareskog et al. 2006).

Inflammation

Inflammation of the synovium is central to the pathophysiology of rheumatoid arthritis, which is characterised by synovitis and joint destruction. Joint erosion results in part from invasion of the joint by proliferating pannus and is mediated by a complex network of interdependent cytokines, most notably interleukin (IL)-1, tumour necrosis factor (TNF)-alpha and IL-6. These cytokines promote inflammation, activate immune cells (including T lymphocytes, B lymphocytes, neutrophils, and mast cells) and non-immune cells (such as fibroblasts and chondrocytes), and lead to the production of injurious mediators such as matrix metalloproteinases (Smolen and Steiner 2003, Tak and Bresnihan 2000). The synovium lining layer hypertrophies and there is infiltration of specific cell types and this is accompanied by new blood vessel formation. Eventual joint destruction, when the condition is not treated, results from the chronic inflammation.

Non-HLA genetic associations with rheumatoid arthritis: loci with strong associations.			
Locus	Protein	Effect	Reference
PTPNN22	Protein tyrosine phosphatase 22	Enhanced regulation of T cell receptor signalling, allowing autoantigen-specific to cells to evade clonal deletion, predisposing to autoimmunity	Vang et al. 2005
TNFAIP3/OLIG3	Tumour necrosis factor, alpha-induced protein 3 and oligodendrocyte transcription factor 3	TNFAIP3: Loss of the NF-κB signalling required for termination of TNF-induced signals (TNF-α levels are raised in RA), chronic inflammation (No musculoskeletal function known for OLIG3)	Plenge et al. 2007
TRAF-1/C5	Tumour necrosis factor associated factor-1 and C5 complement	Propagation of inflammatory response	Barton et al. 2008
STAT-4	Signal transducer and activator of transcription-4		Barton et al. 2008

Figure 1.3 Non-HLA genetic associations with rheumatoid arthritis: loci with strong associations.

Socioeconomic burden of rheumatoid arthritis

Rheumatoid arthritis is a chronic condition, and spontaneous remission in established disease is rare. It classically has its onset during a person's years of peak economic productivity, often between the ages of 30 and 50 with peak onset shortly after (Rindfleisch and Muller 2005). Even with newer treatments, the overall pattern tends to remain one of progression over time, resulting in increased mortality and morbidity; a significant reduction in quality of life as a result of fatigue, pain, and depression; and functional and work disability (Breedveld and Kalden 2004). Furthermore, patients with long-standing rheumatoid arthritis suffer a decrease in socialising activities (Geuskens et al. 2007), although changes over time are generally minor.

Health-care costs

The health-care costs are high (Figure 1.4). Direct health-care costs related to rheumatoid arthritis correlate well with the degree of disability (Figure 1.5). (Fries 1999). For example, a patient with a Health Assessment Questionnaire score of 3 has, on average, three times the health-care costs (at $US 45,000 per patient over 5 years at the time of the study) than a patient with a score of 1. Furthermore, more than 50% of the health-care costs for rheumatoid arthritis are spent on hospital admissions, but these spendings relate to only 10% of patients with rheumatoid arthritis (Yelin and Wanke 1999).

Economic burden for the patient

Other economic costs related to rheumatoid arthritis result from employment changes and restrictions imposed by the pain and disability associated with the condition. The limitations brought about by the disease can result in the need for a change of job or a reduction in work, and in some cases they cause loss of employment or the need for early retirement, all with a consequent reduction in income (Breedveld and Kalden 2004). Employment restrictions often occur early in the course of the disease, and within 2 years of diagnosis, disability benefits are significantly increased, by up to 30% in some study populations (Geuskens et al. 2007). One study of economic burdens that com-

---

Annual health-care costs of rheumatoid arthritis: a US example.

- 250,000 hospital admissions annually (ACR 2002)
- 9 million doctor consultations annually (ACR 2002)
- Medical care costs average $US 6000 for rheumatoid arthritis plus extra $US 2500 for medical reasons not directly related to rheumatoid arthritis. (Yelin and Wanke 1999)
- 50% of the health-care cost is spent on hospital admissions (Yelin and Wanke 1999)

Figure 1.4 Annual health-care costs of rheumatoid arthritis: a US example.

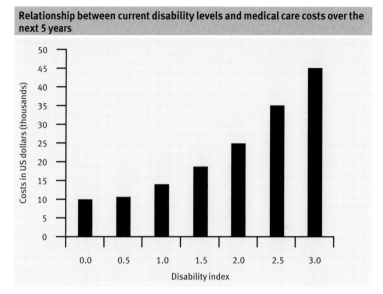

Figure 1.5 Relationship between current disability levels and medical care costs over the next 5 years. Data from Fries 1999.

pared patients with rheumatoid arthritis, osteoarthritis and neither disease noted that patients with rheumatoid arthritis (Gabriel et al. 1997):

- incurred significantly higher expenditures than the control group on such items as home care, child care, home remodelling, and medical equipment and devices;
- had significantly higher burdens than did those with osteoarthritis and were significantly more likely to have lost their job, reduced their working hours, or to have retired early as a result of their illness ($p=0.001$);
- were three times more likely to have had a reduction in their household income than the other groups;
- were more likely to be unable to find work because of their illness (15%, compared with 3% of those with osteoarthritis and 1% of the controls).

Impact of gender and economic status

Women with rheumatoid arthritis are likely to have higher levels of disease activity, to suffer more pain, and to have more significant decline in function and more psychological distress than men (Leeb et al. 2007, Odegård et al. 2007).

Patients in lower income groups tend to be more severely affected than average, in terms of greater disease burden (Harrison et al. 2005, Jacobi et al. 2003, Marra et al. 2004), greater reduction in quality of life (Groessl et al. 2006) and higher mortality (Maiden et al. 1999). This difference may in part be a result of the greater likelihood of delay in specialist rheumatological consultation and poorer medical management overall (Feldman et al. 2007).

Chapter 2

Diagnosis of rheumatoid arthritis

Typical clinical presentation

The typical clinical presentation, in about three-quarters of patients, is one of an insidious onset of joint tenderness and joint swelling. Joint involvement is classically symmetrical, and the small joints of the hands and feet (the meta-carpophalangeal, proximal interphalangeal, and metatarsophalangeal joints) are usually the first to be affected (Suresh 2004). The distal interphalangeal joints are classically spared in rheumatoid arthritis (Figure 2.1). The joints next most commonly involved are the wrists (Boutry et al. 2007). The shoulders and elbows are less commonly affected at the outset, and the hips are rarely involved initially.

Other classic features in the presentation of rheumatoid arthritis include (Suresh 2004):

- **Significant joint stiffness** after periods of inactivity. This is more prominent in the morning and typically lasts for 30 minutes or more on getting out of bed, and may be very prolonged. It is associated with an inability to make a fist or to flex the fingers.
- **Non-specific systemic/constitutional complaints** accompanying the arthralgic features, most commonly a vague feeling of tiredness.

However, there are a number of other ways that rheumatoid arthritis can first manifest itself (Figure 2.2).

Radiological presentation

The classical radiographic changes of rheumatoid arthritis that are seen on plain X-rays, such as peri-articular demineralisation, bony erosions, narrow-ing of the joint space, and ulnar deviation, are not necessarily helpful in early rheumatoid arthritis, since they emerge only once joint destruction has begun and may not be apparent, certainly in very early disease.

Because the initial changes affect soft tissues before affecting bone, ultra-sound and magnetic resonance imaging (MRI) are both more sensitive than

Joints commonly involved in rheumatoid arthritis

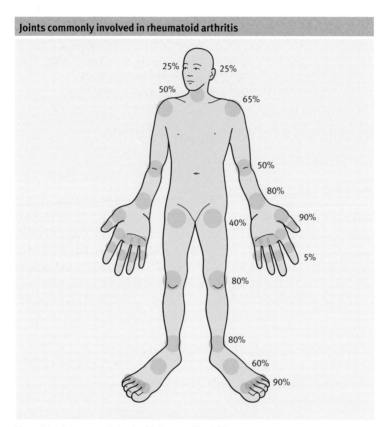

Figure 2.1 Joints commonly involved in rheumatoid arthritis.

Atypical initial manifestations of rheumatoid arthritis

Onset	Characteristics
Monoarticular	Persistent arthritis in a large joint, e.g. knee, shoulder, or ankle
Systemic	Gradual or sudden, with only non-arthritic and non-specific features, e.g. weight loss, fatigue, depression, or fever
Acute polymyalgic	Pelvic or shoulder stiffness of relatively sudden onset, more commonly seen in older people
Palindromic	Repeated episodes of joint pain and swelling involving one or several joints and lasting 1–2 days each time, interspersed with symptom-free intervals; may progress to become a persistent arthritis
Extra-articular (rare)	Vasculitis or serositis

Figure 2.2 Atypical initial manifestations of rheumatoid arthritis. Data from Suresh 2004, Hench and Rosenberg 1944.

Summary of the 1987 ACR criteria for rheumatoid arthritis

Patients must meet four of these seven conditions to fulfil these diagnostic criteria:

- Morning stiffness lasting 1 hour or more that has been present for at least 6 weeks
- Swelling in three or more joints that has been present for at least 6 weeks
- Swelling in the hand joints that has been present for at least 6 weeks
- Symmetrical joint swelling that has been present for at least 6 weeks
- Erosions or decalcification seen on a hand X-ray
- Rheumatoid nodules
- Raised serum rheumatoid factor

Figure 2.3 Summary of the 1987 ACR criteria for rheumatoid arthritis. American College of Rheumatology. Adapted from Arnett et al. 1988.

plain X-rays at detecting early-stage disease (Conaghan et al. 2003a, Sommer et al. 2005, Wakefield et al. 2000). Furthermore, ultrasound detects more erosions of bone than does radiography in the early stages (see Chapter 3). Imaging methods are valuable in establishing a baseline and may be helpful in diagnosing doubtful cases. Imaging in early rheumatoid arthritis is discussed in more detail in Chapter 6.

Diagnostic criteria

A number of diagnostic/classification criteria for rheumatoid arthritis have been devised, the best known of being the American College of Rheumatology (ACR) 1987 Revised Criteria for the Classification of Rheumatoid Arthritis (Figure 2.3) (Arnett et al. 1988).

It should be noted that the ACR criteria, while often used to define rheumatoid arthritis and to distinguish it from other conditions, were developed in populations with long-standing disease and so include chronic manifestations (such as nodules and radiographic erosions) as a means of establishing the diagnosis. They were not designed to detect early disease (Cush 2003). One analysis of the literature published from 1988 to 2006 suggests that the sensitivity and specificity of these criteria to predict rheumatoid arthritis in unclassified early arthritis are 67% and 75%, respectively (Banal et al. 2009). In recognition of this deficiency, a joint ACR/European League Against Rheumatism (EULAR) committee is currently producing new classification criteria.

Differential diagnosis

Distinguishing probable or likely early rheumatoid arthritis from other causes of a patient's symptoms is not always easy. Even if the classic

Differential diagnoses of early rheumatoid arthritis: arthritic signs and symptoms may present in the early stages.

- Post-infective arthritides, which may be viral (e.g. rubella, parvovirus) or occur after a bacterial throat, gastrointestinal, or sexually transmitted infection;

- Connective tissue diseases (e.g. SLE, scleroderma);

- Myalgic disorders (e.g. polymyalgia rheumatica, fibromyalgia);

- Crystal arthropathies (e.g. gout);

- Miscellaneous conditions (e.g. sarcoidosis, thyroid disease, infective endocarditis, paraneoplastic syndromes, multiple myeloma).

Figure 2.4 Summary of the 1987 ACR criteria for rheumatoid arthritis. American College of Rheumatology. Adapted from Arnett et al. 1988.

picture of symmetrical joint involvement is present, the extra-articular manifestations, such as rheumatoid nodules, keratoconjunctivitis sicca, and the pathognomonic radiological changes, are generally absent in early disease. Indeed, extra-articular findings are more likely to appear early in other conditions that have arthritis as a component, for example, the skin and nail manifestations of psoriatic arthritis, the malar rash and serositis of systemic lupus erythematosus, and the lung involvement of sarcoidosis (Dao and Cush 2006).

Other conditions that can present with an early arthritic component are listed in Figure 2.4. Some of the distinguishing features of the common differential diagnoses are listed in Figure 2.5 on pages 12–13.

EULAR recommendations for differential diagnosis

On the basis of expert consensus, EULAR recommends that the differentiation of early rheumatoid arthritis from disorders with similar presentations should involve, at a minimum (Combe et al. 2007):

- a detailed patient history;
- a complete physical examination;
- a full blood count;
- blood tests for transaminases and anti-nuclear antibody;
- a urinalysis; and diagnostic tests (see later).

Other routine tests, depending on the clinical picture, might include uric acid levels, tests for Lyme disease, hepatitis B and C, and parvovirus infection, cultures of urethral or cervical swabs, and anti-bacterial serology.

Diagnostic tests and evaluation of likelihood of progression

There is no single diagnostic test that can establish that a patient has rheumatoid arthritis, and clinical judgement still plays a central role in making the diagnosis in early disease (Härle et al. 2005), which remains largely a clinical skill (NICE 2009). The diagnostic and laboratory tests mentioned above should be performed in all patients who present with symptoms and signs that might be caused by rheumatoid arthritis. Once other diseases have been excluded, the need is to determine which patients are likely to progress to a persistent erosive arthritis, as discussed in Chapter 3.

Differentiating diseases that can present as an early arthritis.

Arthritis	Personal history	Typical pattern of joint involvement	Joints affected	Associated features	Laboratory tests
Undifferentiated arthritis (nonprogressive)	F > M	Insidious Oligoarthritis	PIP, MCP, wrist, MTP, knee, ankle		↑CRP/ESR
Rheumatoid arthritis	F >M 35–50 years	Insidious Progressive Symmetrical	PIP, MCP, wrist, MTP, knee, ankle	EMS	↑CRP/ESR, RF+, CCP+
Spondyloarthropathy	Psoriasis Urethritis or cervicitis, IBD Family history of psoriasis or IBD	Persistent Asymmetric Oligoarticular	DIP, PIP, knee, feet, spine	Psoriasis Nail pitting Uveitis Enthesitis, dactylitis	ESR/ CRP may be normal More severe course in HLA B27 +
Systemic lupus erythematosus	F > M Young	Polyarticular Symmetrical Usually nonerosive	PIP, knee	Rash, serositis	Anaemia, ↑ESR/CRP, proteinuria ANA+, dsDNA+
Viral (HBV, HCV)	Hepatitis risk factors	Acute Polyarthritis	PIP, MCP, wrist, knee, ankles	Jaundice	↑ESR/CRP, ↑LFTs Hepatitis B and C serology
Septic arthritis (nongonococcal)	Peak incidence in elderly Reduced host immunity Joint prostheses	Acute Monoarticular Often extremely painful (Beware may be polyarticular)	Knee – most common Hip, shoulder, ankle, wrist	Systemic symptoms common	Commonest cause: *Staphylococcus aureus* Synovial fluid is gram stain positive in 50% and culture positive in 90%
Gonococcal	F > M Young, sexually active	Acute oligo- or polyarthritis	Wrist, knee	Fever Rash Skin blisters/pustules Tenosynovitis	↑ESR/CRP,↑WBC Synovial fluid gram stain positive in 25% and culture positive in 50% of cases

					Normal laboratory tests
Osteoarthritis	F > M Men with knee or hip involvement ↑Age	Progressive oligo- or polyarticular asymmetric or symmetric, bony sweling	DIP, PIP, CMC1, knee, hip, MTP, spine		
Gout	Men Postmenopausal women Diuretic use (especially in elderly)	Sudden onset, severe pain with attacks oligoarticular early, polyarticular later	MTP, toes, ankle, knees	Tophi	Synovial fluid – urate crystals ↑Uric acid level – (normal levels in 40% of acute attacks)
Pseudogout	M = F ↑Age	Chronic Oligo- or polyarticular Acute monoarticular (25%)	Knee, wrist, finger, MTP	Associated conditions include: Hypomagnesaemia Hypophosphataemia Haemochromatosis Wilson's disease Hyperparathyroidism	↑CRP, ↑WBC
Polymyalgia rheumatica	M = F, Older Caucasian	Prolonged morning stiffness	Hip and shoulder girdle PIP, wrist, knee occasionally	RS3PE	Anaemia, ↑ESR/CRP
Sarcoidosis	F >M	Acute symmetric Chronic uncommon	Knees, ankles	Fever; erythema nodosum and hilar lymphadenopathy with acute sarcoid	↑ESR/CRP Serum ACE
Scleroderma	F > M	Acute or occasionally. insidious symmetric or asymmetric	MCP, PIP Tendon friction rubs (diffuse disease)		↑CRP/ESR ANA +, Scl-70+, ACA+

Figure 2.5 Differentiating diseases that can present as an early arthritis. ACA, anticentromere antibody; ANA, antinuclear antibody; CCP, cyclic citrullinated peptide; CMC1, first carpometacarpal joint; CRP, C-reactive protein; ESR, erythrocyte sedimentation rate; F, female; HBV, hepatitis B virus; HCV, hepatitis C virus; IBD, inflammatory bowel disease; LFT, liver function test; M, male; MCP, metacarpophalangeal joint; MTP, metatarsophalangeal joint; PIP, proximal interphalangeal joint; RA, rheumatoid arthritis; RS3PE, remitting seronegative symmetrical synoritis with pitting oedema syndromeRF, rheumatoid factor; UA, undifferentiated arthritis; WBC, white blood cells. Reproduced with permission from Nam et al. 2007.

Chapter 3

The need for early diagnosis and intervention in rheumatoid arthritis

Until the mid-1980s, the general approach to the treatment of rheumatoid arthritis was to delay the instigation of disease-modifying therapy until the joint erosions became apparent on imaging studies. It was thought that the disease could be controlled with bed rest and aspirin or non-steroidal anti-inflammatory drugs (NSAIDs). However, it began to be realised that any short-term efficacy of these treatments did not translate into long-term disease control. Furthermore, delays in instituting more aggressive treatment with DMARDs and immunosuppressive therapies, rather than protecting patients against their unwanted effect were in fact contributing to increased morbidity and mortality (Pincus and Callahan 1986) in a disease that is chronic and, if not adequately treated, almost always progressive.

Increasingly, evidence has pointed to the importance of the very early use of disease-modifying anti-rheumatic drugs (DMARDs), and it is now well established that aggressive treatment of rheumatoid arthritis early in the disease offers an effective means of slowing disease progression. The fact that erosions are often present at the time of presentation has prompted some authors to conclude that primary care physicians should be motivated to regard early rheumatoid arthritis as a medical emergency, with a view to reducing treatment delays (van der Horst-Bruinsma et al. 1998)

Undifferentiated and early arthritis

However, many patients with early inflammatory arthritis have an undifferentiated arthritis, a form of disease that does not fulfil any criteria for a more definitive diagnosis and for which there are no accepted therapeutic algorithms (Quinn et al. 2003, Verpoort et al. 2004).

The outlook for undifferentiated arthritis ranges from self-limiting disease that remits spontaneously to persistent and erosive disease, including rheumatoid arthritis. One study of several databases noted that the percentage of patients with undifferentiated arthritis that evolved into rheumatoid arthritis within 1 year ranged from 6 to 55%, the large differences between the databases probably being due to differences in the definitions and inclusion criteria used (Verpoort et al. 2004). ACPA positivity in this group increasingly is being regarded as pre-rheumatoid.

If those patients with undifferentiated arthritis who will progress to rheumatoid arthritis can be successfully identified, early treatment can be instigated and disease progression monitored, allowing treatment to be individualised so as to achieve the best possible outcome for each patient.

When rheumatoid arthritis may be classed as 'early' is partly a matter of definition. Results of a survey of European rheumatologists suggested that more than two-thirds consider early rheumatoid arthritis to be disease of 3 months' duration or less. However, the rheumatologists also reported that half of the patients that they see have been referred to them only after 6 months of disease activity (Aleteha et al. 2002), and yet it is estimated that 25% of patients have evidence of erosive disease after 3 months (Breedveld and Kalden 2004) and that 60% have erosive disease after 1 year (Emery et al. 2002).

The problems of early detection

Detection of early rheumatoid arthritis poses a number of difficulties (Suresh 2004) for example:

- **Objective signs of arthritis are not always present**, or they may have been masked or suppressed by NSAIDs.
- **Joint pathology can be difficult to identify** in very early disease, particularly swelling and especially in patients who are obese.
- **Inflammatory markers may not be raised**: in up to 60% patients with early rheumatoid arthritis ESR and CRP are not raised (Emery 1997).
- **Coexisting diseases can complicate the picture** or be confused with rheumatoid arthritis, for example pre-existing osteoarthritis can complicate interpretation of imaging studies, and morning stiffness can also be a feature of osteoarthritis (although it is typically less severe and less prolonged than in rheumatoid arthritis).

The 1987 ACR criteria for rheumatoid arthritis (see Figure 2.3) cannot be entirely relied on for diagnosis in early disease, since they are classification criteria that were developed in populations with established disease and so include chronic manifestations. They have a low sensitivity and specificity for early disease (Banal et al. 2009). As a result of the low sensitivity, patients with early rheumatoid arthritis may not fulfil the criteria and so be misdiagnosed. The low specificity means that

Three steps for evaluation of early arthritis

- **Recognition of presence** of inflammatory arthritis
- **Exclusion of other diseases,** i.e. of diseases other than rheumatoid arthritis or an undifferentiated arthritis that can present with an early inflammatory arthritis (e.g. systemic lupus erythematosus, psoriatic arthritis, spondyloarthropathy)
- **Estimation of risk of progression** to a persistent or irreversible erosive arthritis, by a combination of clinical features, tests, and imaging

Figure 3.1 Three steps for evaluation of early arthritis. EULAR recommendations. [Combe et al. 2007]

patients with other acute but self-limiting conditions, such as post-viral arthritis, may be misdiagnosed and started on inappropriate and aggressive therapy. Thus the ACR criteria should not be relied on as diagnostic tools for early rheumatoid arthritis (Banal et al. 2009, Chogle et al. 1996, Harrison et al. 1998).

The EULAR recommendations are helpful in this regard, suggesting a three-step approach to the evaluation of early arthritis (Figure 3.1) (Combe et al. 2007).

Recognition of the presence of an inflammatory arthritis

Patients who have joint swelling that is not associated with trauma or bony swelling and that is associated with pain or stiffness should be deemed to have arthritis. Anyone who presents with arthritis involving more than one joint for more than 2 weeks should be referred to a rheumatologist and should be seen within 6 weeks of the onset of their symptoms (Combe et al. 2007, Sokka 2008).

The primary method of detecting early arthritis remains clinical examination (Combe et al. 2007) to detect:

- polyarthritis,
- morning stiffness of more than 30 minutes' duration, and
- involvement of the metacarpophalangeal or metatarsophalangeal joints.

Tenderness in a group of small adjacent joints can be assessed by the 'squeeze test' (Figure 3.2), and in single joints it can be determined by isolated gentle palpation of each joint.

ESR and CRP are useful as markers of inflammation, and imaging can be helpful in doubtful cases:

- **Ultrasound (US) and magnetic resonance imaging (MRI)** can be more sensitive than plain radiography in detecting early rheumatoid arthritis (Conaghan et al. 2003a, Sommer et al. 2005, Wakefield et al. 2000) (see Chapters 2 and 6).
- **US and Doppler** may detect synovitis with greater sensitivity than clinical examination by visualising thickened synovial membranes, for example in suspected inflammatory arthritis of the knee (Kane et al. 2003) and erosions (Wakefield et al. 2000).

'Squeeze test' for tenderness in a group of small adjacent joints

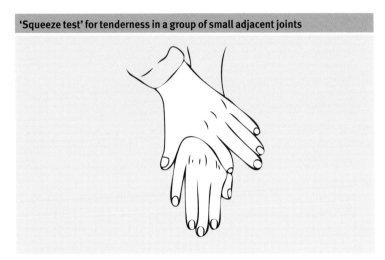

Figure 3.2 **'Squeeze test' for tenderness in a group of small adjacent joints.** This test has been validated for this purpose (Emery et al. 2002, Visser et al. 2002).

- **MRI** may be more sensitive than clinical examination in detecting synovitis and erosions in early rheumatoid arthritis (Forslind et al. 1997, Sugimoto et al. 2000), and these MRI findings may predict subsequent radiological progression (McQueen et al. 2003).

However, the use of these imaging modalities in the diagnosis of rheumatoid arthritis and in predicting likely progression of disease is still at an early stage (Combe et al. 2007).

Exclusion of other diseases

The differential diagnosis of early rheumatoid arthritis is discussed in Chapter 2.

Estimation of the risk of persistence and progression

Once other diseases have been excluded and a diagnosis of rheumatoid arthritis has been established, it is important to be able to identify those patients whose arthritis is likely to persist or progress to erosive disease. This allows progressive disease to be appropriately treated and also avoids unnecessary treatment of non-progressive disease with inappropriate and often toxic therapies. Numerous observational and case–control studies have assessed the prognostic factors in early arthritis or early rheumatoid arthritis. Most of the studies report several independent predictors of long-term radiographic progression of disease:

EULAR recommendations for tests that are predictive of persistent erosive arthritis
• Presence of autoantibodies, including detection of ACPA
• Imaging evidence of bony changes and joint erosions (Visser et al. 2002)
• Presence of IgM or IgA rheumatoid factor (Visser et al. 2002)
• Raised erythrocyte sedimentation rate (ESR) or levels of C-reactive protein (CRP)
• Count of swollen and tender joints (no. of swollen joints probably correlates better with persistent erosive disease than does no. of tender joints (Visser et al. 2002)

Figure 3.3 EULAR recommendations for tests that are predictive of persistent erosive arthritis (Combe et al. 2007). These should be performed once a positive diagnosis has been made.

- the presence of rheumatoid factor,
- a raised ESR or CRP, and
- early radiographic signs of joint erosion.

EULAR recommends that these and the other parameters listed in Figure 3.3 should be assessed as predictive factors. Amongst the laboratory tests, detection of ACPA is the newer method. It is more expensive than measuring rheumatoid factor, which as well as being a relatively cheap test is both diagnostically and prognostically useful in patients with early undifferentiated arthritis (NICE 2009). Indeed, the main value of ACPA is in the early stage of disease when specificity is crucial. However, while ACPA is more specific than rheumatoid factor, the sensitivities of both measures in establishing which patients are likely to progress seem to be very similar (Avouac et al. 2006).

Variables predicting likely persistence of disease in early arthritis and, conversely, a favourable outcome with spontaneous early remission are summarised in Figure 3.4. Duration of symptoms for more than 12 weeks has been suggested to be the most telling predictive factor of all, since spontaneous remission is unlikely in a patient who has had inflammatory arthritic symptoms this long (Green et al. 1999, Suresh 2004).

Evidence from clinical trials to support early intervention

Several randomised controlled trials have shown that early aggressive intervention, allied with careful patient monitoring, is important for achieving the best clinical results and for controlling disease progression.

The evidence is strong in favour of early treatment with DMARDs in patients with arthritis of recent onset. Patients who receive early DMARD treatment have less radiographic progression of disease and better retention of function and ability to work than patients in whom therapy is delayed by only a few months. For example, in a case-control parallel-group study comparing DMARD therapy initiated a median of 3 and 12 months after disease onset, results in favour of

Variables associated with persistence of erosive arthritis and with spontaneous early remission	
Variables predicting persistence of disease[a]	Variables predicting spontaneous early remission
• Autoantibodies, including ACPA • IgM or IgA rheumatoid factor • Imaging evidence of bony changes and joint erosions • Raised acute-phase markers: ESR or CRP • Count of swollen and tender joints • Female sex • Duration of symptoms > 12 weeks • Involvement of joints of hands • History of smoking • Fulfilment of 1974 ACR diagnostic criteria[d]	• Absence of rheumatoid factor[c] • Radiographic evidence of absence of joint erosions[b] • Fewer involved joints[b] • Male sex[b]

[a] Combe et al. 2007, Nam et al. [b] Wolfe and Hawley 1985. [c] Eberhardt and Fex 1998.
[d] Sensitivity 88%, specificity of 73%. CRP, C-reactive protein; ESR, erythrocyte sedimentation rate.

Figure 3.4 Variables associated with persistence of erosive arthritis and with spontaneous early remission.

early therapy [measured by the disease activity score-28, DAS-28 (see Chapter 4), and by assessment of radiological joint destruction using the Larson score] were seen as early as 3 months after initiation (Nell et al. 2004). After 36 months, there was a significant difference in the DAS-28 score improvements (2.8 in the early treatment group versus 1.7 in the later starters, $p<0.05$).

There is also evidence that for patients with undifferentiated arthritis methotrexate may delay the development of rheumatoid arthritis and retard radiological joint damage. In the PROMPT study fewer patients randomised to the methotrexate group progressed to rheumatoid arthritis (40% versus 53%), and patients in the methotrexate group fulfilled the ACR criteria later than did those in the placebo group (Figure 3.5). Similarly, significantly fewer patients in the methotrexate group showed radiological progression over 18 months (12% versus 27%, $p = 0.04$). Among patients with erosions, progression was significantly lower in the methotrexate group than in the placebo group ($p = 0.035$) (Figure 3.6).

It has been suggested that a 'window of opportunity' might exist in rheumatoid arthritis, and in other conditions with an auto-immune component, in which effective treatment can reverse the disease process and prevent the disease from developing (Cush 2007). Even if complete reversal of disease cannot be achieved, therapy during such a window may have a much greater effect than treatment at a later stage in terms of halting progression and achieving remission.

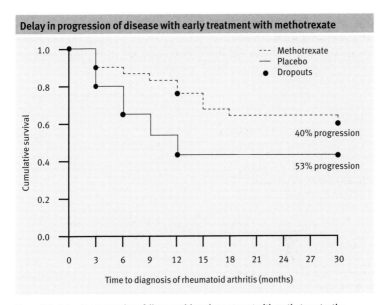

Figure 3.5. Delay in progression of disease with early treatment with methotrexate: the PROMPT study. This study, conducted in The Netherlands from 2001 to 2006, compared 12 months' treatment with methotrexate versus placebo in 110 patients with undifferentiated arthritis. Patients who fulfilled the ACR criteria for rheumatoid arthritis during the course of the 12 months were changed to open-label methotrexate and dropped from the study group (indicated by closed circles). Follow-up was for 30 months. This Kaplan–Meier survival analysis for the diagnosis of rheumatoid arthritis shows that all patients with rheumatoid arthritis in the placebo group who were going to progress to fulfil the American College of Rheumatology criteria had done so within 1 year, compared with only one half of those in the methotrexate group who would eventually progress (p=0.04). Data from van Dongen et al. 2007.

A meta-analysis of 14 randomised controlled trials has confirmed that the best response to DMARDs occurs in patients who are started early on therapy, in this review after less than 1 year of symptoms (Anderson et al. 2000). While other factors that were associated with a better response (male sex, functional class of disease, and disease activity), the strongest indicator was disease duration.

Ongoing clinical trials are studying the window of opportunity in which the consequences of RA can be prevented. For example, one such trial has reported that early treatment with abatacept delayed progression of undifferentiated inflammatory arthritis or very early rheumatoid arthritis in some patients and that the effect continued after cessation of therapy (Emery et al. in press). In this phase II study of 50 patients randomised to 6 months of abatacept or placebo, the modified Sharp radiographic scores and MRI scores for erosion, osteitis and synovitis were better in the abatacept-treated patients at 1 year, with comparable safety in the two groups.

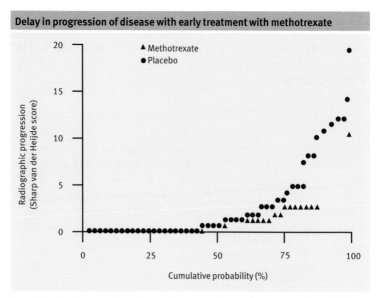

Figure 3.6 Delay in progression of disease with early treatment with methotrexate. Details of the study are given in Figure 3.5. The presence or absence of radiographic progression (using the Sharp/van der Heijde score) at 18 months is shown. Each symbol represents one patient. Data from van Dongen et al. 2007.

Aggressive treatment in early arthritis

Early arthritis clinics

One approach to improving early referral and treatment of rheumatoid arthritis is to use early arthritis clinics, in which patients with possible early disease can be expertly investigated and assessed, treated, and reviewed. Such clinics also aim to identify which patients are likely to develop persistent rheumatoid arthritis (Emery et al. 2002).

The frequent delay in starting treatment has two main causes (Emery et al. 2002):

- delay between symptom onset (which is often insidious) and the patient consulting a primary care physician, and
- delay in making the diagnosis.

Because of the difficulties in making a definitive diagnosis, it is typically the diagnostic delay that is the main factor in the overall delay in starting treatment. It is noteworthy, then, that the effectiveness of early arthritis clinics in making a timely and correct diagnosis in early disease has been demonstrated in a study by van der Horst-Bruinsma et al. (1998). In 70% of patients seen at an early arthritis clinic, a diagnosis of definite rheumatoid arthritis could be made within 2 weeks of the first visit, and the diagnosis, once made, was robust and reliable and was rarely subject to change over the 1-year course of the study.

Nurse-led clinics

Long appointment waiting times in rheumatology services are usually a reflection of a service that is overstretched and also of the need to minimise waiting times for new patients who have possible inflammatory arthritis (Luqmani et al. 2006). Nurse-led clinics can relieve some of the pressure on physician services and facilitate more frequent patient assessment. Usually they are run by rheumatology nurse specialists, who can assess patients with established disease, including:

- monitoring overall health,
- examining joints,
- monitoring of blood tests mandated by therapy, and
- requesting investigations.

In some nurse-led clinics, nurse specialists may also inject joints, prescribe or alter treatments, and carry out therapies such as infusions (NICE 2009).

Outpatient management

Most patients with early rheumatoid arthritis are now treated in outpatient clinics. In the UK in 2007–2008, for example, 93% of rheumatoid arthritis 'patient episodes' were on an outpatient basis, and the change from inpatient- to outpatient-based services has made the acute hospital-based model for rheumatoid arthritis care more economical to run (National Audit Office 2009). Inpatient services are usually reserved for special circumstances, for example day-case intravenous infusion of newer biologic agents or for the patient for whom travel is too difficult for frequent clinic appointments for a specific therapy (SIGN 2000).

Ultimately, the most important factor is not where the care is delivered but rather who delivers it and what is provided, with most units now providing management and patient education via a multidisciplinary team of physicians, specialist nurses, and other health-care professionals (National Audit Office 2009, NICE 2009).

Chapter 4

Treatment of rheumatoid arthritis

Goals of therapy

The goals of therapy in rheumatoid arthritis have been defined as 'symptom control, the reduction of joint damage and disability, and maintenance or improvement of quality of life' (SIGN 2000). In early arthritis, major goals include:

- Control of symptoms and signs of disease, maintenance of function; and fostering of self-efficacy [British Society for Rheumatology guidelines (BSR) (Luqmani et al. 2006)].
- Control of components of disease activity, such as DAS-28 and CRP [NICE guidelines (NICE 2009)].

Both the BSR and NICE guidelines suggest that each patient should be engaged in an individualised care plan that includes an objective measure of disease activity. The ultimate aim of management should be remission of disease (Combe et al. 2007, Luqmani et al. 2006), and, to this end, there is increasing interest in a 'treatment-to-target' approach.

The importance of treatment to target

In many clinical specialties, improvement of outcomes has been facilitated by the adoption of predefined quantifiable treatment targets, for example the haemoglobin A1C level and hypertension control in diabetes. The patient's therapy is adjusted – changing dosage and/or drugs – to achieve the target(s), in a treatment to target approach. In rheumatoid arthritis, assessment of treatment success varies from one institute to the next and there are, as yet, no widely followed guidelines for a 'treatment to target' approach. However, the notion of 'treatment to target' is widely used in clinical trials in rheumatoid arthritis (Strand and Sokolove 2009), allowing and encouraging flexibility in therapeutic regimens to achieve the desired clinical or therapeutic targets.

Historically, complete remission has not always been achievable in practice, because this might require intensive drug interventions to the point of toxicity and medical contact to the point of significant adverse impact on a patient's normal daily activities and psychological state. However, with the introduction of new DMARDs and biologic agents to control inflammation and halt joint damage, remission is now an attainable goal for many patients. Treatment to target has thus become a practical goal for many patients.

One example is a recent 2-year trial of an aggressive 'treatment to target' strategy in early rheumatoid arthritis; it showed that remission can be achieved in about 40% of patients (Goekoop-Ruiterman et al. 2007). The trial therapies were conventional DMARD monotherapies in switching and step-up protocols, and combination therapies consisting of a TNF-α inhibitor plus methotrexate with or without corticosteroids. Patients remained within these groups but, on the basis of 3-monthly assessment of a disease activity score, adjustments were made to the choice of drug(s) from within the drug class. It was noteworthy that the regular monitoring and adjustment of medications meant that all treatment groups achieved almost the same improvement in disease activity and functional ability after 2 years. The trial arms that included a TNF-α inhibitor reduced inflammation more rapidly, reduced disease activity more effectively and had greater structural benefits than those that did not.

Examples of targets that have been suggested for treatment are summarised in Figure 4.1. In practice, the absence of clinical or ultrasound synovitis is not generally achievable with the therapies currently available, and the aim in practice should be to minimise it (Luqmani et al. 2006). Regular monitoring of disease activity should be built into the treatment plan, with escalation of dosage or addition of agents to a combination therapy to reach target. NICE recommends monthly assessments until targets agreed prior to treatment are achieved, and 6-monthly assessments once the disease is under control (NICE 2009).

Measures of disease activity for a 'treatment to target' approach to early arthritis		
Measure	**NICE targets**	**BSR targets**
Composite measure of disease acitivity, e.g. DAS-28 (see Figures 5.1 and 5.2)	Prespecified level agreed with patient	<2.6
C-reactive protein	Prespecified level agreed with patient	Undetectable level
Clinical synovitis		Undetectable level
Ultrasound synovitis		Undetectable level
Reference	NICE 2009	Luqmani et al. 2006

Figure 4.1 Measures of disease activity for a 'treatment to target' approach to early arthritis. BSR, British Society for Rheumatology; DAS-28, Disease activity score-28; NICE, National Institute for Clinical Excellence.

An overview of available medications

The currently available therapies include:

- classical NSAIDs and the newer COX-2 inhibitors,
- corticosteroids,
- conventional DMARDs, often simply called DMARDs, and
- biologic DMARDs ('synthetic' DMARDs or 'biologic agents'), which are divided into the TNF-α inhibitors and agents aimed at targets other than TNF.

NSAIDs and COX-2 inhibitors

Simple analgesics (aspirin or paracetamol) can be effective for pain management in rheumatoid arthritis, but classical NSAIDs and the newer COX-2 inhibitors appear to be more effective in relieving the symptoms and in reducing the signs of active disease (Combe et al. 2007). A significant body of evidence supports this contention, though some of the studies have been conducted in patients with established rheumatoid arthritis rather than early disease (Garner et al. 2002, Wienecke and Gotzsche 2004).

Because of their side-effect profile (see below), the current recommendations are that both COX-2 inhibitors and the older NSAIDs should be used for the shortest possible time and that they should be avoided in those with contraindications to their use. Therefore, while they are valuable agents for symptomatic control in patients with early rheumatoid arthritis, they are not ideal for long-term use and they should be used only after gastrointestinal, cardiac, and renal risk have been evaluated (Combe et al. 2007). It is worth remembering that, in practice, patients with early arthritis have usually been using over-the-counter NSAIDs, before presentation to health-care professionals (Quinn et al. 2003).

Corticosteroids

Corticosteroids have been used to treat rheumatoid arthritis since the 1950s (Hench et al. 1950) and, together with analgesics and anti-inflammatory agents, they were a mainstay of pharmacotherapy until the 1980s. With the advent of the DMARDs and the growing realisation that disease progression can be slowed and remission possibly achieved with more aggressive therapy, the place of corticosteroids in the management of rheumatoid arthritis has become less central and, in some situations, more controversial.

Intramuscular and intra-articular corticosteroids It is undisputed that a single dose of intramuscular or intra-articular corticosteroid is often an effective means of giving rapid symptom relief in very early inflammatory arthritis of less than 12 weeks' duration (Green et al. 1999). Such single-dose therapy can also establish the degree of reversibility of the disease at this early stage, and there is evidence, for example from an open-label study involving 100 patients with early, undifferentiated arthritis, that it might induce remission in some patients (Quinn et al. 2003).

Systemic parenteral corticosteroids as 'bridge therapy' There is also good evidence for such 'bridge therapy' when DMARDs are being started or when their dosage needs to be increased (Choy et al. 1993, Weusten et al. 1993). The doses used may need to be large, and the effects can be expected to last 4–10 weeks, thus providing symptomatic relief before the DMARDs take full effect. Intravenous use may be associated with more severe toxicity than intramuscular use (Weusten et al. 1993).

Long-term use of corticosteroids This is more controversial (Sokka 2008), and long-term high-dose therapy should be avoided because of the risk of side effects (see later). The evidence for any disease-modifying effect is conflicting (Luqmani et al. 2006). The results of several randomised controlled trials (Gotzsche and Johansen 2004) suggest that low-dose oral corticosteroids (typically prednisolone <10 mg/day, or the equivalent) can be effective in relieving short-term signs and symptoms of disease. Some studies suggest that low-dose corticosteroids may have a role in slowing disease progression in the very early stages of the disease (Boers et al. 1997, van Everdingen et al. 2002, Kirwan 1995) but others refute this notion (Capell et al. 2004). It is likely that aggressive step-down combination regimens with DMARDs are the most effective , as shown by the COBRA study, which demonstrated that an initial period of combination of prednisolone and methotrexate with sulphasalazine continued to have benefits during 4- to 5-year follow up despite withdrawal of the corticosteroid methotrexate (Boers et al. 1997, Landewe et al. 2002).

DMARDs

DMARDs have been used for more than 40 years, but before the 1980s they were rarely used in early rheumatoid arthritis; when they were, the preparation was usually intramuscular gold (Sokka et al. 2008). As strong evidence has accumulated in favour of early initiation of DMARDs in patients with early rheumatoid arthritis, they are now the cornerstone of management. Prompt institution of DMARD therapy is key to successful management, and patients with early arthritis who are at risk of developing a persistent or erosive arthritis should be started on DMARDs as soon as possible, whether or not they fulfil one of the formal classification criteria for rheumatoid arthritis or another inflammatory arthritic condition (Nam et al.).

The 'conventional' or 'synthetic' DMARDs are listed in Figure 4.2. Since the 1990s, methotrexate has become in practice the first-line DMARD in the treatment of rheumatoid arthritis (Klaukka and Kaarela 2003, Sokka et al. 1997, Sokka et al. 2008). The advantages of methotrexate include:

- its relatively better adverse-effect and safety profile compared with other conventional DMARDs;
- its record of clinical and radiological efficacy; and
- beneficial properties when used as part of combination therapy with biologic agents.

Recent evidence-based recommendations from the ACR provide detailed guidance about the choice of DMARDs in different patient groups. In early rheumatoid arthritis, the recommendations are that (Saag et al. 2008):

- methotrexate, leflunomide, or sulphasalazine are suitable as monotherapy for patients regardless of disease activity and prognosis;
- hydroxychloroquine can be used as monotherapy in patients who do not have poor prognostic features;
- methotrexate plus hydroxychloroquine as dual therapy is recommended for patients with moderate or high disease activity;
- methotrexate plus leflunomide as dual therapy is recommended for patients with high disease activity and disease duration of more than 6 months.

Toxicity and side effects from DMARDs and patient monitoring are discussed later. Although DMARDs are potentially toxic agents, the risks from the DMARDs in current use are less than the risks of severe problems developing from inadequately treated rheumatoid arthritis (Möttönen et al. 2002). Nevertheless, the DMARDs do not produce satisfactory outcomes in all patients, and in one study of patients with very early rheumatoid arthritis given DMARDs when the duration of symptoms was less than 3 months, 64% had developed erosive disease by 3 years (Machold et al. 2007).

'Conventional' or 'synthetic' disease-modifying antirheumatic drugs (DMARDs)		
Commonly used	**Infrequently used**	**Rarely used**
Methotrexate	Hydroxychloroquine/chloroquine	Cyclosporin
Leflunomide	Injectable gold	Auranofin
Sulphasalazine	Azathioprine	Cyclophosphamide

Figure 4.2 'Conventional' or 'synthetic' disease-modifying antirheumatic drugs (DMARDs).

TNF-α inhibitors for rheumatoid arthritis

TNF-α inhibitor	Action	Dosage	Methotrexate co-therapy
Etanercept	Recombinant human TNF-α-receptor fusion protein Binds to TNF-α and blocks TNF-α lymphotoxin and competitive inhibitor	25–50 mg s.c. twice weekly	Co-prescribe unless MTC not tolerated or not appropriate
Infliximab	Chimeric monoclonal antibody Binds soluble and transmembrane TNF-α with high affinity and inhibits binding of TNF-α to cell-surface TNF receptors	3 mg/kg i.v. over 2 hours at weeks 0, 2 and 6, and thereafter every 8 weeks Dose or frequency can be increased if response not adequate	Essential to co-prescribe
Adalimumab	Human-sequence antibody, binding TNF Binds soluble and transmembrane TNF-α and inhibits binding of TNF-α to cell-surface TNF receptors Changes biological responses induced by TNF-α, e.g. levels of adhesion molecules responsible for leukocyte migration	Combination therapy: 40 mg s.c. fortnightly Monotherapy: up to 40 mg weekly	Co-prescribe unless MTX not tolerated or not appropriate
Certolizumab	Recombinant, humanised antibody Fab' fragment against TNF-α Binds soluble and transmembrane TNF-α and, because lacks Fc portion, does not bind complement or lyse cells that have transmembrane TNF-α	Combination therapy: 400 mg s.c. (divided into two 200 mg doses on a single day) in weeks 0, 2 and 4, then 200 mg s.c. every 2 weeks Monotherapy: as for combination therapy	Co-prescribe unless MTX not tolerated or not appropriate

Figure 4.3 TNF-α inhibitors for rheumatoid arthritis. Each drug is licensed for active RA in adults when response to conventional DMARDs (including MTX) is inadequate, and in severe active progressive RA in adults not previously treated with MTX. DMARD, disease-modifying antirheumatic drug; MTX, methotrexate; RA, rheumatoid arthritis; TNF-α, tumour necrosis factor alpha. Data from NICE (2009), Barnes and Moots (2007), and Summary of Product Characteristics for Cimzia (certolizumab.

Biologic agents

Biologic agents provide potent anti-inflammatory effects, modifying disease processes, and have been used in early arthritis.

TNF-α inhibitors

TNF-α is a cytokine that is key to the inflammatory cascade and has an important role in the persistence of early rheumatoid arthritis (Nam et al.). Currently, four TNF-α inhibitors are licensed for treating rheumatoid arthritis (Figure 4.3). Several randomised controlled trials have looked at the effects of TNF-α inhibitors in early disease, as discussed below.

Comparisons with methotrexate

One study that compared monotherapy with etanercept (10 mg or 25 mg twice weekly) versus monotherapy with methotrexate in patients with early erosive arthritis of less than 3 years' duration found that overall response during the first 6 months (assessed using a measure of the reduction in the number of tender and swollen joints) was significantly higher in patients receiving the higher dose of etanercept than in those receiving methotrexate monotherapy (Bathon et al. 2000).

Another study compared the clinical and radiological outcomes in patients with early, aggressive disease (of less than 3 years' duration), who received monotherapy with either twice-weekly intramuscular etanercept (10 or 25 mg) or oral methotrexate (mean dose 19mg per week) for 2 years (Genovese 2002). The study was double-blinded for the first 12 months, after which patients went on to receive their study medication for the next 12 months in an open-label manner. Radiologists assessing the X-ray findings remained blinded throughout. The study concluded that etanercept as monotherapy was superior to methotrexate as monotherapy in terms of decreasing disability, reducing disease activity, and arresting structural damage over the 2 years of the trial.

Combination therapy

More studies have looked at combination therapy with a biologic therapy plus methotrexate (Breedveld et al. 2006, Quinn et al. 2005, St Clair et al. 2004). These have also shown a higher rate of clinical remission and slowing of radiographic changes in patients receiving combination therapy than in patients receiving methotrexate alone.

One study looked at a subgroup of patients who had not shown clinical improvement (as measured by the ACR 20% criteria) in 54 weeks of therapy on either infliximab (3 mg/kg or 10 mg/kg every 4 or 8 weeks) plus methotrexate or on methotrexate plus placebo (Smolen et al. 2005). Despite the less than optimum clinical response in all the patients included in the study, those receiving combination therapy showed slower radiological progression of disease than those receiving methotrexate alone ($p<0.05$ to <0.001).

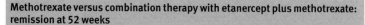

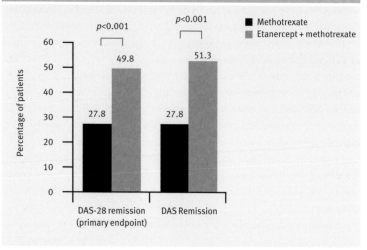

Figure 4.4 Methotrexate versus combination therapy with etanercept plus methotrexate: remission at 52 weeks. Adapted from Nam et al. 2007, based on data from Emery et al. 2008a.

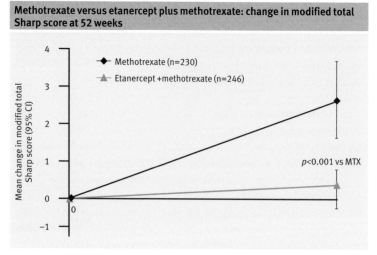

Figure 4.5 Methotrexate versus combination therapy with etanercept plus methotrexate: change in modified total Sharp score (TSS) at 52 weeks. Adapted from Nam et al. 2007, based on data from Emery et al. 2008a.

Combination therapy with remission as a primary end-point

As mentioned earlier, clinical remission and radiological non-progression may well be achievable goals in patients with early rheumatoid arthritis, including those patients at the more severe end of the disease spectrum.

The COMET study was the first major trial to look at remission (defined as a DAS-28 score <2.6 – see Figures 5.1 and 5.2) as a primary end-point in patients with early moderate or severe rheumatoid arthritis (Emery et al. 2008a). 542 patients with symptoms of less than 2 years' duration and who had not previously received methotrexate were randomised to receive methotrexate (titrated from 7.5 mg to a maximum of 20 mg per week by week 8) as monotherapy or methotrexate plus etanercept (50 mg per week). Significantly more patients who received the combined therapy achieved remission at 1 year, (Figure 4.4). The combination group also had a higher rate of radiological non-progression (measured with the modified total Sharp score) than the methotrexate group (Figure 4.5). The rate of serious adverse events, serious infections, and malignancy was similar between the two groups.

Speed of clinical response

Studies of infliximab (St Clair et al. 2004), etanercept (Bathon et al. 2000), and adalimumab (Breedveld et al. 2006) also suggest that the TNF-α inhibitors, whether used alone or in combination therapy, produce a more rapid clinical response than methotrexate alone in early rheumatoid arthritis. One study that compared infliximab (3 or 6 mg/kg) plus methotrexate versus methotrexate alone in patients with early rheumatoid arthritis who had not received methotrexate before found that more patients in the infliximab group had clinically meaningful improvement in Health Assessment Questionnaire (HAQ) scores and that this difference was seen as early as week 2 of treatment. Similarly, rapid and sustained improvement in health-related quality of life, fatigue and other patient-reported outcomes were found in a randomized controlled comparison of certolizumab plus methotrexate and placebo plus methotrexate (Strand et al. 2009). Reductions in fatigue, disease activity, pain and physical dysfunction were reported at week 1.

A three-way comparison of adalimumab plus methotrexate versus adalimumab alone versus methotrexate alone in patients with early disease (less than 3 years' duration; mean 0.7 years), similarly showed that the combination therapy in early disease produced rapid disease control and better clinical outcomes than when either was used as monotherapy (Breedveld et al. 2006). ACR 50% improvement criteria were achieved in 61% of the patients receiv-

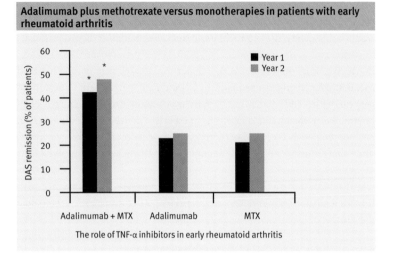

Adalimumab plus methotrexate versus monotherapies in patients with early rheumatoid arthritis

The role of TNF-α inhibitors in early rheumatoid arthritis

Figure 4.6 Adalimumab plus methotrexate versus monotherapies in patients with early rheumatoid arthritis. * p<0.001 versus adalimumab alone and versus methotrexate alone. MTX, methotrexate. Data from Breedveld et al. 2006.

ing combination therapy compared with 42% of those receiving adalimumab monotherapy and 46% of those receiving methotrexate monotherapy (both *p*<0.001). Clinical remission defined as a DAS-28 <2.6 after 1 and 2 years was significantly better with adalimumab plus methotrexate than with either drug alone (Figure 4.6). There was also significantly less radiographic progression with combination therapy at 1 year (1.3 Sharp units) than with adalimumab alone (3.0 Sharp units) or methotrexate alone (5.7 Sharp units) (*p* ≤ 0.002).

The role of TNF-α inhibitors in early rheumatoid arthritis

The studies described above demonstrate that the TNF-α inhibiting biologic agents, generally in combination with methotrexate:

- enable more rapid control of inflammation than with a DMARD alone,
- allow earlier remission to be achieved than is achieved with a DMARD alone, and
- are more likely to limit structural joint damage.

They are therefore particularly useful for patients who will not have a good response to monotherapy with a DMARD. The problem with this approach is that it is not possible to predict accurately which patients will not respond to DMARDs alone.

Moreover, the cost of the TNF-α inhibitors, which are significantly more expensive than the older DMARDs, limits their use in practical terms for many patients, particularly in early rheumatoid arthritis, since the benefits have not yet been shown to outweigh the financial costs. The cost–benefit balance would be changed if they could be used exclusively in high-risk patients likely to respond to treatment (Ikeda et al. 2007). Better still would be the situation in which poor prognosis could be predicted at a stage before a diagnosis of rheumatoid arthritis can be made. This would allow treatment to be started very early, even perhaps within the 'window of opportunity' for prevention of progression to rheumatoid arthritis suggested by Cush (2007). So far, however, evidence has not been found to correlate treatment outcome with any patient or disease characteristics or genetic or other factors (Ikeda et al. 2007).

The conventional DMARDs and the newer biologic agents are not optimally effective in all patients. Newer biologic agents that have been used in established rheumatoid arthritis are being tried in early disease, and new biologic therapeutic modalities are being developed, as discussed below.

Biologic agents aimed at targets other than TNF

A number of biologic agents aimed at targets other than TNF are licensed for treatment of patients with rheumatoid arthritis in whom therapy with conventional DMARDs or TNF-α inhibitors has failed:

- rituximab,
- abatacept, and
- tocilizumab.

Studies are currently underway to assess their potential as disease-modifying treatments in early RA. At present, however, clinical trial data are available only in the setting of established RA.

There have been no head-to-head comparisons of efficacy and safety of the available biologic DMARDs (Singh et al. 2009). At present there is thus no knowledge as to whether any particular biologic agent is more effective and safer for any one subgroups of patients with RA.

Rituximab

Rituximab is a monoclonal antibody directed against the CD20 surface antigen on B cells. It causes a rapid and significant decrease in synovial B cell numbers (Vos et al. 2007). The diminution of both peripheral and synovial B cells is variable, however, and this variability is thought to be related to levels of clinical response (Dass et al. 2008, Kavanaugh et al. 2008).

Rituximab has been used as monotherapy or in combination with another agent such as methotrexate or cyclophosphamide (Edwards et al. 2004).

NICE recommends its use in combination with methotrexate for severe active rheumatoid arthritis in adults who have responded inadequately to or are intolerant of other DMARDs (including at least one TNF inhibitor) (NICE 2009). Its efficacy in long-standing RA (c. 12 years in duration) in this setting was demonstrated in the Randomized Evaluation of Long-Term Efficacy of Rituximab in RA (REFLEX) Trial, a phase III study of rituximab plus methotrexate versus placebo plus methotrexate. At 24 weeks, rituximab plus methotrexate produced significant and clinically meaningful improvements in disease activity (Figure 4.7). Swollen and tender joint counts, disease activity, pain scores, disability scores, CRP levels, and ESRs were significantly decreased. There were also significant reductions in fatigue and joint-space narrowing, and a non-significant trend to less radiographic evidence of joint damage (Cohen et al. 2006). Recently the first evidence has been published to show that in patients with long-standing active RA, an inadequate response to a TNF inhibitor and receiving methotrexate, rituximab significantly reduces radiographically evident progression of joint damage (Keystone et al. 2009).

Rituximab has also been studied in combination with corticosteroids in patients with established RA. In the phase IIb Dose-Ranging Assessment: International Clinical Evaluation of Rituximab in Rheumatoid Arthritis (DANCER) trial, significantly more patients who received rituximab plus corticosteroid therapy met the ACR 20% improvement criteria and achieved moderate or good EULAR response than did patients receiving placebo plus corticosteroid therapy (Emery et al. 2006).

Abatacept

Abatacept inhibits T-cell function by blocking T-cell activation. Studies have found it to be effective in the management of rheumatoid arthritis that has not responded adequately to either methotrexate or TNF-α inhibitors (Kremer et al. 2005). A number of trials have found it to be more effective in combination with methotrexate than as monotherapy (Donahue et al. 2008), and its license is for use in this combination in severe active rheumatoid arthritis in adults who have responded inadequately to or are intolerant of other DMARDs (including at least one TNF inhibitor).

In the USA, abatacept has recently also been licensed for use in patients with moderate-to-severe rheumatoid arthritis of ≤ 2 years duration, on the basis of results from the Abatacept study to Gauge Remission and Joint Damage Progression in Methotrexate-Naïve Patients with Early Erosive Rheumatoid Arthritis (AGREE) trial. In this trial, significantly more patients who were taking

Responses to treatment at week 24 in the REFLEX trial comparing rituximab with placebo

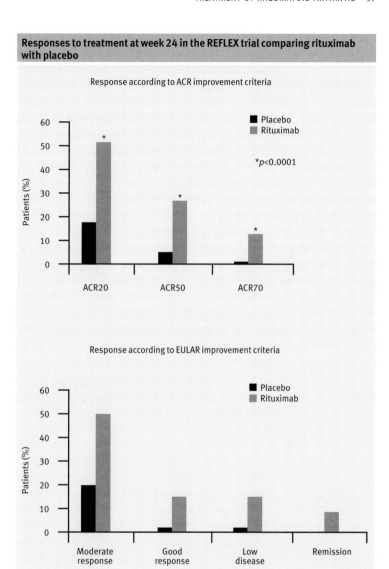

Figure 4.7 Responses to treatment at week 24 in the REFLEX trial comparing rituximab with placebo. EULAR responses are: moderate, DAS-28 <5.1 and an improvement of 0.6–1.2; good, DAS-28 <3.2 and an improvement of >1.2; low disease activity, DAS-28 ≤3.2; remission, DAS-28 <2.6. ACR, American College of Rheumatology; EULAR, European League Against Rheumatism; REFLEX, Randomized Evaluation of Long-Term Efficacy of Rituximab in RA. Data from Cohen et al. 2006.

abatacept plus methotrexate had a good activity score (DAS-28-CRP < 2.6) than did those on methotrexate alone, and significantly more achieved ACR 20, 50 and 70% improvement at 3, 6 and 12 months (Full prescribing information, 2009).

On cost-effectiveness grounds, in the UK abatacept is not currently recommended for the treatment of rheumatoid arthritis (NICE 2008, 2009). Furthermore, although abatacept is usually well tolerated, there have been questions about its safety profile, particularly in combination therapy (Weinblatt et al 2006).

As mentioned earlier, clinical data published to date on the newer biologic agents have been in the setting of established disease rather than very early rheumatoid arthritis. However, an ongoing phase II study of the impact 6 months treatment of abatacept in undifferentiated inflammatory arthritis or very early rheumatoid arthritis has recently been reported (Emery et al. in press). At 1 year, 6 months after cessation of treatment, radiographic and MRI scores were better in abatacept-treated patients than in the placebo-treated group, with comparable safety in the two groups.

Tocilizumab

Tocilizumab is a monoclonal antibody that targets the IL6-receptor (Ohsugi and Kishimoto 2008). It has been found to be effective in rheumatoid arthritis that is resistant to treatment with conventional agents, and it has been licensed for use in this indication.

In one of the earliest trials of tocilizumab in patients with active rheumatoid arthritis and an inadequate response to methotrexate, at 16 weeks the percentage of patients achieving the ACR 20% improvement criteria was higher for the group taking tocilizumab alone and for the group taking tocilizumab with methotrexate than was the case for patients on methotrexate monotherapy (Maini et al. 2006). More recent trials have confirmed this result in patients with moderate to severe active rheumatoid arthritis (Smolen et al. 2008), including trials in patients with an inadequate response to one or more TNF-α inhibitors (Emery et al. 2008b). In the largest trial to date, of 1220 patients with active rheumatoid arthritis, the ACR20% response was achieved in 61% of the group receiving tocilizumab plus a conventional DMARD and 25% of the group receiving only a conventional DMARD ($p< 0.0001$) (Genovese et al. 2008). Secondary endpoints, including ACR50, ACR70, DAS-28 and EULAR responses, and markers such as C-reactive protein and haemoglobin levels also demonstrated the superiority of tocilizumab plus DMARDs versus DMARDs alone.

A benefit in terms of radiographic evidence of structural joint damage has also been demonstrated for tocilizumab. At the end of a 1-year study of patients with active rheumatoid arthritis of < 5 years duration, the tocilizumab monotherapy group had significantly less radiographic change in Sharp score than did the conventional DMARD group [mean 2.3 (95% CI 1.5–3.2) vs. mean 6.1 (95% CI 4.2–8.0), p< 0.01] (Nishimoto et al. 2007).

Other biologics in development

A number of other biologics are in development. These include additional TNF inhibitors (golimumab) as well as agents targeting CD20 (ocrelizumab, ofatumumab, TRU-015), lymphotoxin pathways (briobacept) and other B-cell targets, including BLyS and APRIL (belimumab, atacicept). (Bingham 2008).

Conservative vs aggressive treatment approaches

The days when a conservative treatment approach could be considered a good standard of care for early rheumatoid arthritis are in the past. Up until the early 1990s, many patients with rheumatoid arthritis were treated with only NSAIDs and perhaps low-dose corticosteroids until there was radiological evidence of joint damage (Weinblatt 2004). Now, however, early use of a DMARD and sometimes a biologic agent is the norm. Recent trials support aggressive treatment as the more effective option in patients with early rheumatoid arthritis as a means of slowing disease progression (Ikeda et al. 2007), and a strong recommendation of the BSR guidelines is that that patients with early rheumatoid arthritis should be started on disease-modifying therapy as soon as possible after a diagnosis of rheumatoid arthritis is established (Luqmani et al. 2006). Such therapy should be part of an aggressive package of care, which may entail:

- escalating doses of therapeutic agents;
- use of intra-articular steroid injections;
- parenteral methotrexate; and
- combination therapy, rather than sequential monotherapy, progressing to the use of biologic agents (anti-TNF-alpha) when required.

Overview of safety and tolerability profiles

NSAIDs and COX-2 inhibitors

Traditional NSAIDs, particularly in long term use, are associated with side effects, most notably gastrointestinal complications, but they also carry renal and cardiovascular risks. The concomitant use of gastroprotective agents (such as proton pump inhibitors, misoprostol, or H2-blockers) (Combe et al. 2007, Rostom et al. 2003), and use of enteric-coated formulations of NSAIDs, substantially reduce the risk of gastrointestinal complications, especially gastric bleeding.

COX-2 inhibitors were developed in part to have a better side-effect profile than the older NSAIDs, and they carry a lower risk of bleeding and other gastrointestinal effects. However, there are concerns about their adverse cardiovascular risk profile, as noted in the EULAR recommendations (Combe et al. 2007) and elsewhere, adverse effects that are probably shared to an extent with the traditional NSAIDs.

Corticosteroids

The risk of adverse effects with corticosteroids is dependent both on the dose used and the condition being treated, and it may be that the fears in rheumatoid arthritis are overestimated, probably because of an emphasis on reports from high-dose therapy (Da Silva et al. 2006). Nevertheless, side effects remain a potential problem:

- The cumulative effects of corticosteroid therapy in the long term need to be borne in mind (Luqmani et al. 2006).
- Long-term therapy (prednisolone >10 mg/day, or equivalent, for more than a few weeks) should be avoided (Sokka 2008).

Musculoskeletal effects: osteoporosis is probably the most common adverse effect of longer-term use of corticosteroids. A review of clinical trials looking at the safety of corticosteroids in rheumatoid arthritis (Da Silva et al. 2006), suggested that bone mineral density (BMD) is little different in patients with rheumatoid arthritis treated with low-dose corticosteroids and those receiving placebo. In the four main trials, the dose was ≤10 mg/day of prednisolone or the equivalent. However, one of these trials did find that the incidence of radiographic vertebral fractures in the corticosteroid group was twice that in the placebo group, although the different was not statistically significant (van Everdingen et al. 2002).

Osteoporosis can be prevented or minimised by therapies to prevent or treat bone loss (Figure 4.8).

The data on osteonecrosis are less clear, but it is generally accepted that it is uncommon in patients taking low-dose corticosteroids (Da Silva et al. 2006). Nevertheless, a high index of suspicion should be maintained.

Weight and body fat: redistribution of body fat, a known complication of long-term high-dose corticosteroids, is also observed with lower doses. Weight gain with central obesity but sparing of the limbs is the hallmark. Weight gain can also be a feature of lower-dose therapy: a review of four studies (Da Silva et al. 2006) found that low-dose oral corticosteroid therapy over 2 years was associated with a mean increase in body weight of 4–8%, and in two of the studies the increase in weight was significantly more than in the placebo patients.

Prevention and treatment of corticosteroid- associated osteoporosis

- Concomitant therapy:
  - Recommended: concomitant supplementation with calcium and either vitamin D or an activated form of vitamin D (e.g. alfacalcidiol or calcitriol) to restore calcium balance and maintain bone mass
  - If appropriate: bisphosphonates to prevent and treat bone loss
- Therapy should be continued as long as the patient is receiving corticosteroids (American College of Rheumatology 2001)

Figure 4.8 Prevention and treatment of corticosteroid- associated osteoporosis.

Hormonal effects: high-dose corticosteroids have effects on sex hormone secretion, for example lowering levels of oestrogen and testosterone (Da Silva et al. 2006) These changes are the result of central effects on the hypothalamus and pituitary and a decrease in responsiveness of gonadal tissues to luteinising hormone. Nevertheless, it appears that there may be no clinically relevant effect on fertility in patients being treated for rheumatoid arthritis with low-dose therapy, and spontaneous patient complaints of decreased libido appear to be uncommon.

Cardiac effects of corticosteroids include accelerated atherosclerosis, allied with dyslipidaemia, an increase in blood pressure, and cardiac failure. They are dose-related and less likely with current regimens used in the management of rheumatoid arthritis (Da Silva et al. 2006). Increased susceptibility to infection is similarly less likely with low-dose or sporadic use of corticosteroids, as are the diabetogenic effects, but any patients taking long-term or high-dose corticosteroids should have regular blood glucose testing.

Conventional DMARDs

Regular monitoring of adverse events, together with the patient response, should guide decisions on choice and changes in treatment strategies (Combe et al. 2007). Adverse events of the most commonly used DMARDs in rheumatoid arthritis, together with recommended routine monitoring, are summarised in Figure 4.9.

Infection: methotrexate and leflunomide should not be started in patients with active bacterial infection, active or latent tuberculosis, active herpes zoster, or life-threatening fungal infections (Saag et al. 2008). They can be started shortly after a bacterial infection has resolved or been successfully treated with antibiotics. DMARDs should probably not be started in the presence of severe upper respiratory tract infections (whatever the aetiology) or in patients with unhealed infected skin ulcers. Methotrexate should be avoided in patients

Profile of some commonly used DMARDs in rheumatoid arthritis

Drug	Common or minor adverse events	Rare or severe adverse events	Contraindications and cautions	Monitoring	Advantages
Methotrexate	Nausea, diarrhoea Mouth ulcers Rash, alopecia Abnormal liver function tests	Leukopenia, thrombocytopenia Pneumonitis, sepsis Liver disease Epstein–Barr virus-associated lymphoma	Acute bacterial or life-threatening fungal infection, latent or active tuberculosis, active herpes zoster infection Low leukocyte or platelet count Myelodysplasia or recent lymphoproliferative disease (≤5 years) Abnormal liver function tests, hepatitis B, hepatitis C Renal impairment (reduce dose); pregnancy or breast-feeding	Full blood count, liver function tests, renal function tests Advice to limit alcohol	Rapid onset of action (6–12 weeks) Can be used even when diagnosis is uncertain Weekly administration, and can be given orally, intramuscularly, or subcutaneously
Sulphasalazine	Nausea, diarrhoea Headache Mouth ulcers Rash Reversible oligospermia Abnormal liver function tests	Leukopenia	Abnormal liver function tests, hepatitis B, hepatitis C Pregnancy or breast-feeding	Full blood count, liver function tests, renal functions; urinalysis	Rapid onset of action (8–12 weeks) Can be used even when diagnosis is uncertain Relatively safe in thrombocytopenia
Leflunomide	Alopecia Diarrhoea, nausea Rash	Leukopenia, thrombocytopenia Hepatitis	Acute serious bacterial or fungal infection, latent tuberculosis Low leukocyte or platelet count Myelodysplasia or recent lymphoproliferative disease (≤5 years)	Full blood count, liver function tests, renal function tests; blood pressure	Still to be determined

| Hydroxychloroquine | Nausea Headaches | Retinal toxicity | Abnormal liver function tests, hepatitis B, hepatitis C Pregnancy or breast-feeding | Hepatitis B, hepatitis C Retinal impairment (reduce dose) Pregnancy or breast-feeding | Eye check | No blood monitoring needed Can be used even when diagnosis is uncertain Can be used despite leukopenia or thrombocytopenia |

Figure 4.9 **Profile of some commonly used DMARDs in rheumatoid arthritis.** DMARD, disease-modifying anti-rheumatic drug. Adapted from SIGN and Saag et al. 2008.

with pneumonitis associated with rheumatoid arthritis or in patients with interstitial lung disease of unknown cause.

Methotrexate and leflunomide should not be started or re-started in patients with a leukocyte count <3000/mm^3, and methotrexate, leflunomide, and sulphasalazine are contraindicated if the platelet count is <50,000/mm^3 (Saag et al. 2008). Myelodysplasia or recent lymphoproliferative disease are also contraindications for the use of methotrexate and leflunomide.

Before commencing therapy with a DMARD, vaccinations are recommended against (Saag et al. 2008):

- influenza for treatment with methotrexate, leflunomide, sulphasalazine, or hydroxychloroquine;
- *Streptococcus pneumoniae* for treatment with methotrexate, leflunomide, or sulphasalazine;
- hepatitis B for treatment with methotrexate or leflunomide.

Hepatic and renal disease: methotrexate, leflunomide, and sulphasalazine should not be started or re-started when liver transaminase levels are above twice the upper limit of normal (Saag et al. 2008). These agents are also contraindicated in active hepatitis B or hepatitis C infection and should be used with caution in patients with chronic infection.

Methotrexate is contraindicated in patients with renal impairment and a creatinine clearance <30 ml/minute.

Pregnancy and breast-feeding methotrexate and leflunomide should not be used in pregnancy or in patients who are planning pregnancy, and they should be avoided during breast-feeding.

Circumstances in which DMARDs should be withdrawn: DMARDs may need to be stopped or the dosage reduced in patients with early rheumatoid arthritis in the event of the development of significant adverse effects or intercurrent illness. It is also recommended that they be withdrawn during the perioperative period in patients undergoing surgery, for at least 1 week before and 1 week after the operation (Saag et al. 2008). Patients in whom DMARDs must be stopped should have arrangements in place for early review (NICE 2009).

Biologic agents

TNF-α inhibitors are generally well tolerated and have a good safety profile, but important adverse events have been reported (Breedveld and Kalden 2004), in particular:

- opportunistic infection, including tuberculosis,
- malignancy,
- demyelinating disorders,
- a lupus-like syndrome, and
- congestive heart failure.

Because of concerns about adverse events, patients should be evaluated carefully before commencing treatment with TNF-α inhibitors, to rule out contraindications (Figure 4.10) and to obtain information relating to the potential for adverse events (Figure 4.11). Vigilance for potential adverse events should be maintained throughout the course of therapy. In particular monitoring for infections, notably for TB, should continue during therapy and it should be continued for 5–6 months after therapy because elimination of TNF-α inhibitors takes up to 6 months.

Adverse events associated with TNF-α inhibitors are discussed in more detail below. There has been less experience with biologic agents aimed at targets other than TNF (rituximab, abatacept, tocilizumab). However, as they too are immunomodulatory agents, there are similar concerns relating to raised risk of serious infections and malignancy. Absolute contraindications to their use are listed in Figure 4.12.

Infection The risk of serious infections in patients with RA treated with TNF-α inhibitors is increased compared with placebo. One meta-analysis obtained an odds ratio of 2.0 (95% CI, 1.3–3.1) (Bongartz et al. 2006).

In particular, registry data from several countries have reported an increased risk of tuberculosis with TNF-α inhibitors. For example, in a comparison of 3106 patients taking DMARDs with 10,403 patients in the BSR Biologics

---

Contraindications to use of TNF-α inhibitors

- Hypersensitivity to the active substance or to any of the excipients (and, for infliximab, to other murine proteins)
- Active tuberculosis
- Other acute severe bacterial, fungal and viral infections
- Active chronic or localised infections, especially hepatitis B
- Treated lymphoproliferative disease of <5 years
- Multiple sclerosis or other demyelinating disorder
- Moderate or severe heart failure (NYHA class III/IV)

Figure 4.10 Contraindications to use of TNF-α inhibitors. Data from Saag et al. 2008, Summary of Product Characteristics for Embrel (etanercept), Summary of Product Characteristics for Humira (abatacept), Summary of Product Characteristics for Remicade (infliximab).

Checklist for evaluation and vaccination of patients before commencing TNF-α inhibitors for the treatment of rheumatoid arthritis	

Patient evaluation	• Rule out infections in general
	• Evaluate for both active and latent tuberculosis:
	  ◊ Detailed history of tuberculosis and/or exposure to tuberculosis
	  ◊ Previous and/or current immunosuppressive therapy
	  ◊ Tuberculin skin test and chest X-ray
	• Obtain full blood count, liver transaminases and creatinine
	• Evaluate risk of hepatitis B infection or reactivation
	• Examine for signs of non-melanoma skin cancer
	• Evaluate risk of heart failure

Vaccination	• *Streptococcus pneumoniae* • Influenza • Hepatitis B, if risk factors are present • Live vaccinations are contraindicated
Action if TB is diagnosed	• Active TB rules out initiation of biologic agents • Latent ('inactive') disease mandates anti-tuberculosis treatment prior to initiation of biologic, under the guidance of a physician with expertise in tuberculosis treatment

Figure 4.11 Checklist for evaluation and vaccination of patients before commencing TNF-α inhibitors for the treatment of rheumatoid arthritis. Data from Saag et al. 2008, Summary of Product Characteristics for Embrel (etanercept), Summary of Product Characteristics for Humira (abatacept), Summary of Product Characteristics for Remicade (infliximab).

Contraindications to the use of biologic agents aimed at targets other than TNF
• Hypersensitivity to the active substance or to any of the excipients (all) or to murine proteins (rituximab) • Active, severe infections (all) • Severe heart failure (New York Heart Association Class IV) or severe, uncontrolled cardiac disease (rituximab)

Figure 4.12 Contraindications to the use of biologic agents aimed at targets other than TNF (rituximab, abatacept, tocilizumab). Data from Summary of Product Characteristics for MabThera (rituximab), Summary of Product Characteristics for Orencia (abatacept), Summary of Product Characteristics for RoActemra (tocilizumab).

Registry (BSRBR) who were taking TNF-α inhibitors, TB was diagnosed only in anti-TNF treated patients and occurred at significantly higher rates with infliximab and adalimumab than with etanercept (Dixon et al. 2008).

Malignancy There are concerns that the risk of malignancy, including lymphoma and skin cancer, can be increased with TNF-α inhibitors. This is biologically plausible, given that TNF-α (as its full name suggests) has a role in the prevention of tumorigenesis. However, investigation of this issue is complicated by the fact that rheumatoid arthritis itself increases the rate of malignancy (Chakravarty and Genovese 2004) and by the difficulties posed by the relatively small size and short time span of randomized controlled trials of biologics: individual trials have been insufficiently powered to assess rare and long-term side effects.

Whilst meta-analyses and large observational studies might be expected to circumvent these problems, it has been noted that they have produced contradictory results in general (Nasir and Greenberg 2007). For example, in a meta-analysis Bongartz et al. (2006) found that, compared with control treatment, the pooled odds ratio of malignancy (all types) with infliximab and adalimumab was 3.3 (95% CI 1.2–9.1). In contrast, in the same year a cohort study pooling US and Canadian databases concluded that users of biologic agents were unlikely to have a substantial increase in haematological malignancies or solid tumours (Setoguchi et al. 2006).

Problems in the study by Bongartz et al. (2006) were subseqeuntly identified, including an unexpectedly low incidence of malignancy in the control arm (possibly following detection and drop-out during pre-trial screening) and the fact that the increased risk was mostly found at doses higher than those usually used in the clinic (Dixon and Silman 2006). It is noteworthy, then, that a more recent meta-analysis found that with recommended doses of TNF-α inhibitors there were no increases in the odds ratios (ORs) of lymphoma (OR 1.26; 95% CI 0.52– 3.06), non-melanoma skin cancers (OR 1.27; 95% CI 0.67–2.42) or the composite endpoint of non-cutaneous cancers plus melanomas (OR 1.31; 95% CI 0.69–2.48) in exposure-unadjusted evaluations, with similar results after adjustment (Leombruno et al. 2009).

Further difficulties in analysing trial and registry date relate to the choice of comparator in the latter type of study and, in both types, to the long time period over which malignancy develops. Askling et al. (2009) found that, compared with patients newly starting methotrexate, those newly starting TNF-α inhibitors had no increase in the risk of malignancy of [relative risk (RR) 0.99, 95% CI 0.79–1.24]. Restricting the comparison to only those patients who were on the early rheumatoid arthritis register gave a similar result (RR 0.96, 95% CI 0.64–1.42). Comparison of patients taking TNF-α inhibitors and biologic-naïve patients also showed no increased risk (RR 1.00, 95% CI 0.87–1.17) and the RR did not change with increasing cumulative time on TNF-α inhibitors; furthermore, beyond the first year, no differences were observed between the three drugs.

In the same comparison of patients taking TNF-α inhibitors and biologic-naïve patients, exclusion of non-melanoma skin cancer (NMSC) did not appreciably alter the RRs (Askling et al. 2009). However, TNF-α inhibitors have been associated with an increased risk in comparison with conventional DMARDs of developing non-melanoma skin cancer (NMSC), particularly basal and squamous cell skin cancers. For example, in a retrospective cohort study of 16,829 patients from the US Department of Veterans' Affairs database, 3096 of whom were on TNF-α inhibitors, those on TNF-α inhibitors had a higher risk of developing NMSC (hazard ratio 1.34, 95% CI 1.15–1.58; p<0.0001), with an incidence of 25.9 per 1000 patient-years (Amari et al. 2009). Similarly, Wolfe and Michaud (2007) found an increased risk for NMSC and melanoma during 49,000 patient years in the US National Data bank for Rheumatic Diseases.

Thus, whilst further research is undoubtedly required to establish definitively whether biologic agents increase the rate of malignancy, in the meantime it is advisable to maintain a high index of suspicion for malignancy during treatment with biologic agents, especially when other risk factors are present, including risk factors for skin cancer.

Demyelinating neuropathy This is a rare adverse event of treatment with TNF-α inhibitors. However it usually improves over a period of months after treatment withdrawal and/or in association with immunomodulating treatments for neuropathy control (Lozeron et al. 2009, Stübgen 2008).

Anti-TNF-induced lupus (ATIL) Although TNF-α inhibitors are commonly associated with the induction of autoantibodies, ATIL is rare. Its frequency and clinical characteristics vary between different drugs, however withdrawal of therapy usually leads to resolution of ATIL symptoms (Williams et al. 2009).

Congestive heart failure There have been rare reports of worsening congestive heart failure (CHF) without identifiable precipitating factors in patients with rheumatoid arthritis who are taking TNF-α inhibitors. Cardiovascular risk is increased in rheumatoid arthritis, concomitant with inflammation and raised levels of circulating cytokines. Theoretically, then, TNF inhibition should reduce heart failure risk in rheumatoid arthritis by reducing inflammation. However, despite suggestions that this is the case (Listing et al. 2008), currently the direction of their impact on cardiovascular risk in RA is unknown (Gabriel 2008).

Pregnancy Data from one of the world's largest registries (BSRBR) have shown a trend towards a higher rate of miscarriage in women taking TNF-α inhibitors at the time of conception than in those who had previously ceased taking the therapy (King et al. 2008). Thus TNF-α inhibitors cannot be advocated during pregnancy until further studies have confirmed their safety.

Chapter 5

Monitoring disease progression, treatment response and outcome

Regular monitoring of disease activity should be used to guide decisions on choice of treatment and the need for changes in treatment strategies (Combe et al. 2007). Various measures are used to assess the progression of rheumatoid arthritis and treatment responses, usually in combination. They include:

- counts of clinically affected joints,
- laboratory tests,
- clinical measures, such as morning stiffness and grip strength, and
- radiographic measures.

Joint count measures

As well as being good predictors of the likelihood of persistence of disease in early undifferentiated arthritis, joint counts are also used to monitor progression and treatment responses. They are included in most scoring systems [e.g. the DAS-28 (van Riel and Schumacher 2001); see Figures 5.1 and 5.2], and

---

Disability activity score-28 (DAS-28)

DAS-28 is a composite score, calculated from:

- Number of swollen joints — 'swollen-28' — and the number of tender joints — 'tender-28' — assessed using counts from 28 specific joints: shoulders, elbows, wrists, metacarpophalangeal joints, proximal interphalangeal joints and knees
- Erythrocyte sedimentation rate (ESR, in mm/hour)
- An assessment of either general health (GH) or global disease activity made by marking a 10 cm line to indicate a level between 'very good' and 'very bad'

The formula used for calculating DAS-28 is:

DAS-28 = [0.56 × √(tender28)] + [0.28 × √(swollen28)] + [0.70 × ln(ESR)] + [0.014 × GH]

Figure 5.1 Disability activity score-28 (DAS-28). Adapted from information on the website of the Department of Rheumatology, University Medical Centre, Nijmegen, The Netherlands (http://www.das-score.nl/www.das-score.nl/)

Joints assessed in the disease activity score-28 (DAS-28)

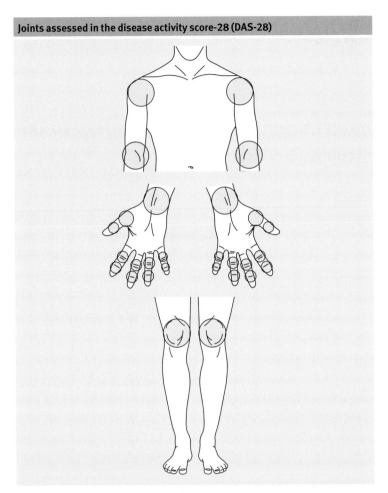

Figure 5.2 Joints assessed in the disease activity score-28 (DAS-28). Adapted from information on the website of the Department of Rheumatology, University Medical Centre, Nijmegen, The Netherlands (http://www.das-score.nl/www.das-score.nl/)

they form part of the criteria that have been devised to assess improvement (Felson et al. 1995, van Gestel et al. 1996) and remission (Pinals et al. 1981, Prevoo et al. 1996).

Other measures include a patient count of joints that are painful, and a count of joints in which there is limitation or pain on movement. It can be useful to use a cartoon showing the major joints for documenting disease (Figure 5.3).

Cartoon for documenting pain, swelling and deformity during follow up of rheumatoid arthritis

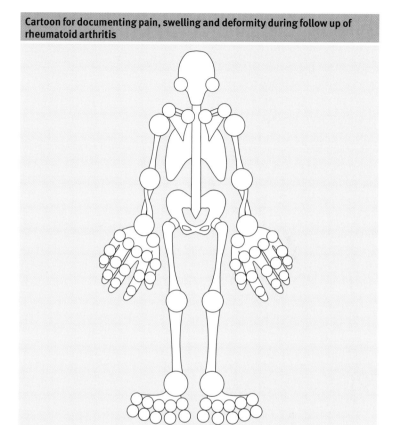

Figure 5.3 Cartoon for documenting pain, swelling and deformity during follow up of rheumatoid arthritis.

Laboratory measures

Although the presence of rheumatoid factor in a patient with early undifferentiated arthritis is predictive of progression to rheumatoid arthritis, and is a good predictor of prognosis (NICE 2009, Nam et al.), it is not as good a measure of response to treatment as other laboratory measures, including acute-phase reactants (ESR and CRP) and haemoglobin levels.

A normochromic, normocytic or microcytic anaemia is typically seen in rheumatoid arthritis (about 25% of patients respond well to iron therapy). In those with an anaemia of chronic disease, the haemoglobin level tends to correlate well with the ESR, and change in haematological parameters is a good surrogate measure of response to treatment (Rindfleisch and Muller 2005).

Clinical measures

Morning stiffness in a patient with early undifferentiated arthritis is a good predictor of persistence (van der Helm-van Mil et al. 2007b, Visser et al. 2002) and points to rheumatoid arthritis as a likely diagnosis (Arndt et al. 2007). In patients with early inflammatory arthritis, it has been suggested that a history of ever having had morning stiffness is more predictive of rheumatoid arthritis than is currently having it (El Miedany et al. 2006).

Grip strength can be measured using a blood pressure cuff inflated to about 30 mmHg. The patient is then asked to squeeze the cuff as hard as possible. The test can be repeated for each hand, and the score can be recorded as the mean of the results (Pincus et al. 1994).

Walking tests are also useful: the patient is timed while walking a certain distance (typically 25 feet or about 7.5 m) (Kazis et al. 1990). This test can be extended by asking the patient to get up out of a chair before the walk and to sit down in a chair at the end of it (Pincus et al. 1994).

Radiographic measures

Early radiographic evidence of erosions predicts long-term radiographic progression. Erosions occur earlier in the course of rheumatoid arthritis than was once supposed, and recent studies suggest that more than 80% of patients have evidence of erosions within the first 2 years (Combe et al. 2007), and nearly 50% of patients can develop erosions within the first year (Fex et al. 1996).

Plain radiography is the most commonly used means of assessing joint damage in rheumatoid arthritis. Other changes of early rheumatoid arthritis that can be visualised on imaging include hyperaemia (associated with acute inflammation and occurring in exacerbations of established disease as well as early arthritis), synovitis, effusions, and narrowing of the joint space. Subluxation, luxation, and joint destruction are features more likely to be seen in advanced disease.

Imaging techniques in rheumatoid arthritis are discussed in more detail in Chapter 6.

Criteria for remission of rheumatoid arthritis

Rheumatoid arthritis is a life-long disease and, although combination therapy with DMARDs and biologic agents can lead to some remission in up to 40% of patients, significant disease generally persists (Olsen and Stein 2004; Pincus et al. 1999) and complete remission is rare. Various criteria for remission have been used. Each set of criteria includes some requirement that there should be

Summary of the ACR remission criteria

At least five of the criteria must be met:
- Morning stiffness lasting less than 15 minutes
- No fatigue
- No joint pain at rest
- No joint tenderness or pain on motion
- No soft tissue swelling
- Erythrocyte sedimentation rate < 20 mm/hour in men, < 30 mm/hour in women

Figure 5.4 Summary of the ACR remission criteria. ACR, American College of Rheumatology. Adapted from Pinals et al. 1981.

a lack of clinical evidence of disease activity and that progression of disease should have been arrested (NICE 2009). The ACR criteria for remission are shown in Figure 5.4. Remission has also been defined as a DAS score <1.6 or a DAS-28 score <2.6 (Prevoo et al. 1996).

Fulfilment of formal remission criteria does not guarantee true disease-free status. Recent studies have shown that most patients who would be classed as being in remission have synovitis that can be detected on imaging, indicative of continuing subclinical inflammation. For example, in one study of patients on DMARDs and in clinical remission on DMARDs, MRI showed evidence of synovitis in 96% and bone marrow oedema in 46%, and ultrasound revealed synovial hypertrophy in 73% (Brown et al. 2006). In a subsequent study of patients in remission, 19% showed deterioration in radiographic joint damage over 12 months (Brown et al. 2008).

This continuing subclinical inflammation in patients in clinical remission may account for the discrepancy that has been noted between apparent disease activity and outcome. In the future, imaging may be necessary for the accurate evaluation of disease status and remission criteria may need to be developed that take imaging status into account (Brown et al. 2006).

Recommendations for monitoring treatment response

Patients who have been diagnosed with rheumatoid arthritis require regular reviews so that treatment can be modified as needed (National Audit Office 2009). NICE guidance suggests that monitoring should be monthly in early rheumatoid arthritis and that this frequency should be maintained until the disease is controlled by treatment (NICE 2009). The frequency of further monitoring can be decided on an individual basis to suit each patient.

The NICE guidance also recommends an annual review with the aim of:
- assessing disease activity and measuring functional ability,
- checking for the development of co-morbidities,

- assessing symptoms that suggest that complications are developing,
- organising appropriate cross-referral within the multidisciplinary team of health-care providers,
- assessing any need for referral for surgery, and
- assessing the effect that the disease is having on the patient's life.

Response to treatment can be measured against criteria developed by the ACR and EULAR. The ACR improvement criteria were developed for use in clinical trials and define clinical response as a percentage improvement in a number of measures (Figure 5.5) (Felson et al. 1995). The EULAR criteria divide patients into three groups according to changes in the DAS score (Figure 5.6) (van Gestel et al. 1996). One major difference of this system from the ACR criteria is that it takes into account absolute current disease activity as well as improvement.

Summary of the ACR response criteria

Improvement is measured in terms of percentage improvement (20, 50 or 70%):
- Improvement in number of tender joints
- Improvement in number of tender and swollen joints
- Improvement in three of five measures:
  - Global assessment by the patient (using a 10 cm visual analogue scale, ranging from 'disease not active at all' at zero to 'disease very active' at 10)
  - Global assessment by the physician or other investigator
  - Pain as assessed by the patient
  - Health Assessment Questionnaire or another score of physical disability
  - Erythrocyte sedimentation rate or C-reactive protein

Figure 5.5 Summary of the ACR response criteria. Adapted from Felson et al. 1995. ACR, American College of Rheumatology.

Summary of the EULAR response criteria

Patients are divided into three groups on the basis of their DAS score:

1. Good responders
Patients with > 1.2 improvement from baseline DAS or DAS-28 plus DAS ≤ 2.4 or DAS-28 ≤ 3.2 at endpoint

2. Moderate responders
Patients with > 0.6 but > 1.2 improvement from baseline DAS or DAS-28 plus DAS > 2.4 but ≤ 3.7 or DAS-28 > 3.2 but > 5.1 at endpoint

3. Non-responders
Patients with ≤0.6 improvement from baseline DAS or DAS-28 plus DAS > 3.7 or DAS-28 > 5.1 at endpoint

Figure 5.6 Summary of the EULAR response criteria. EULAR, European League Against Rheumatism. Adapted from van Gestel et al. 1996.

Chapter 6

Imaging techniques in rheumatoid arthritis

Imaging plays a key role in both the diagnosis and the ongoing assessment of rheumatoid arthritis. Plain radiographs, particularly of the hands and feet, have been used in the diagnosis and evaluation of rheumatoid arthritis (Sokka 2008) and in differentiating it from other conditions associated with arthritis (Sommer et al. 2005). Longitudinal studies have generally used radiographic progression as a means of tracing the natural history of the disease and its possible modifications by therapy.

What techniques are available?

The imaging modality that has traditionally been used to assess joint disease in rheumatoid arthritis is of course the plain X-ray. Plain X-rays, particularly of the hands and feet, have been used in the evaluation of rheumatoid arthritis for at least the past 60 years, and it was largely long-term cohort studies using radiographic evaluations and comparisons that led to the realisation of the destructive nature of the disease (Sokka 2008, Sommer et al. 2005).

However, in early rheumatoid arthritis the changes are not bony, and therefore ultrasound and magnetic resonance imaging (MRI) are both better than plain X-rays at detecting disease in the early stages (Conaghan et al. 2003a, Sommer et al. 2005, Wakefield et al. 2000):

- **Ultrasound** using high-resolution probes is limited to superficial joints, and it can be difficult to obtain reliable images of weight-bearing surfaces or joint surfaces that are shadowed by overlapping bone (McQueen and Ostergaard 2007).

- **Power Doppler ultrasound** may be useful in assessing disease activity (Sommer et al. 2005), but its utility has not been fully established (Wamser et al. 2003) and the available data are sparse.

- **MRI** is currently the best means of detecting damage to the soft-tissues, and it is moreover superior to both plain X-rays and ultrasound at showing changes in cartilage and bone.

In practical terms, both MRI and ultrasound are less readily available and more costly than plain X-rays (Sokka 2008), and MRI is significantly more time-consuming to perform, an issue for staffing and costs and also for patients who are having frequent imaging investigations. As a result, plain X-rays continue to be widely used for the assessment of joint changes in rheumatoid arthritis as well as for the monitoring of disease progression and the response to treatment.

Computed tomography (CT) is rarely used, since it is not as good as MRI at detecting changes in rheumatoid arthritis and it carries the disadvantage of subjecting the patient to radiation. It has little place in the assessment and management of early disease.

Assessing radiographic progression

There is no general consensus on which joints should be imaged. For the purposes of diagnosis, any joint that is clinically affected should be imaged, as should the joints typically involved in rheumatoid arthritis (the joints of the hands and wrists and probably the joints of the feet) (Sommer et al. 2005). Some of the scoring methods for radiological joint disease in rheumatoid arthritis specify which joints should be imaged for the purposes of calculating the score (e.g. the Sharp method), though others do not (e.g. the Larson method).

When plain X-rays are used, it is important that optimal resolution is ensured. In most centres, a certain number of joints are imaged at standard intervals in order to follow patients. The joints imaged would usually include any symptomatic joints as well as the joints of the hands, feet, and cervical spine, and possibly others.

In MRI, axial and sagittal images should be performed on the basis of coronal images in order to define the pathological changes. A multiplanar approach can be useful in distinguishing between erosions and pre-erosive changes (Sommer et al. 2005). T1-weighted images with and without contrast, a T2-weighted image, and images that can visualise cartilaginous changes should be performed.

MRI protocols usually involve imaging of one or both hands as typical early sites for rheumatoid arthritis, and most MRI scoring systems are based on findings in the hands and wrists (Sommer et al. 2005). There are some variations in scoring even between experienced assessors, however levels of agreement in scoring erosions, synovitis and edema are considered acceptable, and agreement between assessors is better for metacarpophalangeal joints than for wrists (Conaghan et al. 2003b).

Joint abnormalities

A number of abnormalities at an affected joint can be seen on imaging (Sommer et al. 2005):

- **Hyperaemia** is the first change that can be seen by imaging. Although there are usually no changes on plain radiography, it can be seen on Power Doppler ultrasound with contrast and on MRI (Stone et al. 2001, Wamser et al. 2003).

- **Synovitis** can be detected by ultrasound (Figure 6.1) and by MRI (Figure 6.2) before it becomes clinically apparent (Conaghan et al. 2004). However, imaging changes of mild synovitis are also sometimes seen in the joints of healthy subjects, which suggests that an imaging finding of synovitis in a clinically normal joint may have a lower than ideal specificity (Combe et al. 2007).

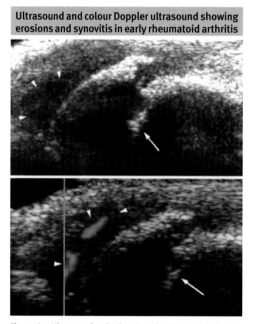

Ultrasound and colour Doppler ultrasound showing erosions and synovitis in early rheumatoid arthritis

Figure 6.1 Ultrasound and colour Doppler ultrasound showing erosions and synovitis in early rheumatoid arthritis. The gray-scale longitudinal ultrasound image shows thickened hypeochoic synovium (arrowheads) in the second metacarpophalangeal joint (A). In the power Doppler longitudinal ultrasound image, there is marked Doppler signal (4+) present in the synovium (arrowheads) and a punctate Doppler signal arising within the depth of the erosion, consistent with infiltrating pannus (arrow). Reproduced with permission from Bajaj S, Lopez-Ben R, Oster R, Alarcón GS. Ultrasound detects rapid progression of erosive disease in early rheumatoid arthritis: a prospective longitudinal study. Skeletal Radiol 2007 Feb;36(2):123-8.

MRI showing synovitis in early untreated rheumatoid arthritis

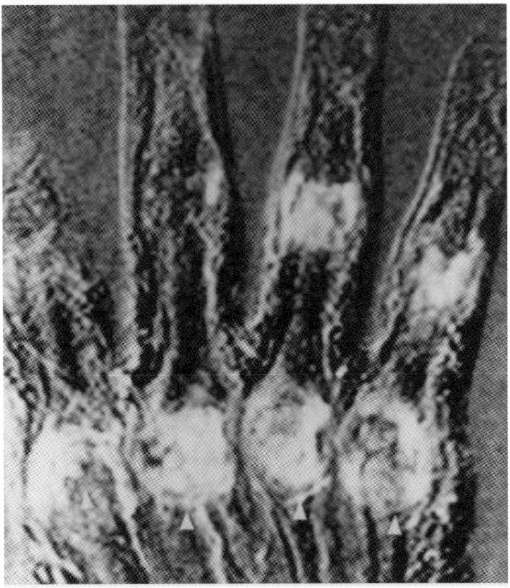

Figure 6.2 MRI showing synovitis in early untreated rheumatoid arthritis. A spoiled gradient-echo subtraction gadolinium-diethylenetriaminepentaacetic acid (Gd-DTPA) pulse sequence was used to show synovitis. In this patient, prominent Gd-DTPA enhancement is evident in the second to fifth metacarpophalangeal joints (arrowheads). Reproduced with permission from McGonagle D, Conaghan PG, O'Connor P, et al. The relationship between synovitis and bone changes in early untreated rheumatoid arthritis. A controlled magnetic resonance imaging study. Arthritis Rheum 1999;42:1706–1711.

- **Joint effusions** are revealed better by ultrasound and MRI than by plain radiography (Figure 6.3) (Sommer et al. 2005).
- **Narrowing of the joint space** is reasonably readily seen on plain X-rays (Figure 6.4). With the advent of newer imaging modalities and the increased emphasis on very early identification of rheumatoid arthritis, it is no longer regarded as a marker of early disease (Nam et al., Sommer et al. 2005). It is caused by destruction of the cartilage, and in rheumatoid arthritis it is usually concentric in nature (in contrast to the narrowing seen in osteoarthritis, which is typically uneven in nature). It is one of the parameters assessed in the commonly used scoring methods for radiological changes in rheumatoid arthritis.
- **The presence of erosions** is commonly used for quantitative assessment of joint involvement. MRI is the modality that can identify erosions at

Erosion at the metacarpophalangeal joint in early rheumatoid arthritis

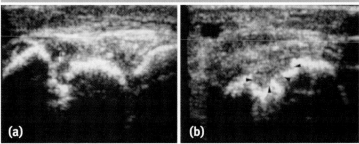

Figure 6.3 Erosion (arrows) at the metacarpophalangeal joint in rheumatoid arthritis.
Longitudinal (a) and transverse (b) views are shown. Reproduced with permission from
Wakefield RJ, Kong KO, ConaghanPG, et al. The role of ultrasonography and magnetic
resonance imaging in early rheumatoid arthritis. Clin Exp Rheumatol 2003;21:S42–S49.

Plain radiograph showing joint-space narrowing in early rheumatoid arthritis

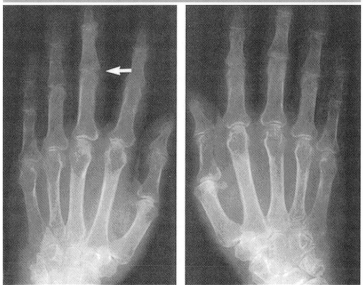

Figure 6.4 Plain radiograph showing joint-space narrowing in early rheumatoid arthritis.
As well as diffuse periarticular osteopenia and early joint-space narrowing in the wrist,
erosions are evident at the margins of the joints (e.g. left third proximal interphalangeal
joint, arrow). Courtesy of Gilliland B, Wener M. Atlas of Infectious Diseases: Skin, Soft
Tissue, Bone, and Joint Infections. Edited by G Mandell (series editor), TP Bleck. Current
Medicine Group, 1995.

Direct comparison of radiography and MRI in visualising erosions in early rheumatoid arthritis

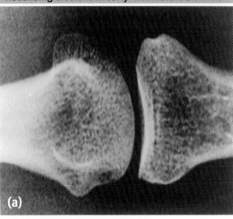

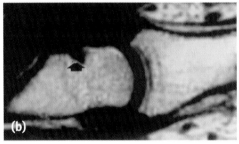

Figure 6.5 Direct comparison of radiography and MRI in visualising erosions in early rheumatoid arthritis. The radiograph shows normal results for this second metacarpophalangeal joint (a) whereas the T1-weighted spin-echo pulse sequence) coronal demonstrates an erosion on the radial aspect of the second metacarpal (b). MRI, Magnetic resonance imaging. Reproduced with permission from Wakefield RJ, Gibbon WW, Conaghan PG, et al. The value of sonography in the detection of bone erosions in patients with rheumatoid arthritis. A comparison with conventional radiography. Arthritis Rheum 2000;43:2762–2770.

the earliest stage (Figure 6.5). In one study of 42 patients, erosions were identified at the wrist in 45% of the patients 4 months after the onset of symptoms, a stage when only 15% had erosions that were detectable on plain X-rays (Figure 6.4).

- **Late changes in advance disease**, such as destruction of the peri-articular structures, fibrosis, subluxation, and ankylosis.

Quantitative analysis of radiographs

Methods of analysing radiographs quantitatively to assign a score to the imaging findings have been widely used for research purposes, both to trace the course of the disease over time in cohorts and to assess the effects of treatment strategies in slowing progression. They also have some utility in managing the treatment of individual patients.

The first methods to be used to score radiographs in rheumatoid arthritis were the Steinbrocker and the Kellgren method. Both scored damage to joints in the hands and the wrists. The most widely used methods have been the scoring systems developed by Larsen and by Sharp in the 1970s (Larsen et al. 1977, Sharp et al. 1971), both of which have been subsequently modified. These scales each assess two joints on scales of zero to 5 at each joint, on the basis of:

- erosions
- joint-space narrowing

The Sharp method uses separate scores for these, while the Larsen method is based on a global score for each joint. The Sharp system scores a defined selection of joints, whereas all synovial joints can be included in the Larsen score and therefore the joints that are scored should be listed with it.

Further modifications of the Sharp score have been developed. The best known is probably that developed by van der Heijde to produce the Sharp–van der Heijde score (SHS) (van der Heijde 1999b; van der Heijde et al. 1999c). The erosion score in the SHS is calculated by looking at 16 areas of each hand and wrist, and at each side of the 10 metatarsophalangeal joints and two intra phalangeal joints in the feet.

These methods are useful for research purposes, with the Larsen method being more easily scored and less time-consuming than the Sharp method (Sokka 2008), but they are complicated to learn and relatively difficult to use. This limits their usefulness in the ordinary clinical setting. A more practical scoring method for ordinary use may be the Simple Erosion Narrowing Score (SENS), which is a simplified adaptation of the SHS (van der Heijde 2000). It combines the two abnormalities assessed in the SHS – erosions and narrowing of the joint space – on a zero to 2 scale. The same joints are assessed as in the SHS. Comparisons between the SHS and the SENS show similar utility for clinical use in early rheumatoid arthritis (van der Heijde 2000).

Regardless of which scoring method is used, the initial score at the time of diagnosis is a consistent predictor of the future radiological damage (Jansen et al. 2001).

Chapter 7

Guidelines

The EULAR recommendations for the management of early arthritis were published in 2007 (Combe et al. 2007). The steering group consisted of 14 rheumatologists from 10 European countries. A total of 15 issues were selected for further research by the group, which based its recommendations on the available evidence as at January 2005 and on expert opinion. The guidelines contain 12 key recommendations for the management of early arthritis, including early rheumatoid arthritis:

- Arthritis is characterised by the presence of joint swelling, associated with pain or stiffness. Patients presenting with arthritis of more than one joint should be referred to, and seen by, a rheumatologist, ideally within 6 weeks of symptom onset.
- Clinical examination is the method of choice for detecting synovitis. In doubtful cases, ultrasound, power Doppler, and MRI might be helpful.
- Exclusion of diseases other than rheumatoid arthritis requires careful history taking and clinical examination, and ought to include at least the following laboratory tests: full blood cell count, urinanalysis, transaminases, and antinuclear antibodies.
- In every patient presenting with early arthritis to the rheumatologist, the following factors predicting persistent and erosive disease should be measured: number of swollen and tender joints, ESR or CRP, levels of rheumatoid factor and ACPA, and radiographic joint erosions.
- Patients who are at risk of developing persistent or erosive arthritis should be started with DMARDs as early as possible, even if they do not yet fulfil established classification criteria for inflammatory rheumatological diseases.
- Patient information concerning the disease and its treatment and outcome is important. Education programmes aimed at coping with pain, disability, and maintenance of the ability to work may be used as adjunct interventions.

- NSAIDs have to be considered in symptomatic patients after evaluation of gastrointestinal, renal, and cardiovascular status.
- Systemic corticosteroids reduce pain and swelling and should be considered as adjunctive treatment (mainly temporary), as part of the DMARD strategy. Intra-articular corticosteroid injections should be considered for the relief of local symptoms of inflammation.
- Among the DMARDS, methotrexate is considered to be the anchor drug, and should be used first in patients at risk of developing persistent disease.
- The main goal of DMARD treatment is to achieve remission. Regular monitoring of disease activity and adverse events should guide decisions on choice and changes in treatment strategies (DMARDs here including biologic agents).
- Non-pharmaceutical interventions such as dynamic exercises, occupational therapy, and hydrotherapy can be applied as adjuncts to pharmaceutical interventions in patients with early arthritis.
- Monitoring of disease activity should include tender and swollen joint count, patient's and physician's global assessments, ESR, and CRP. Arthritis activity should be assessed at intervals of 1–3 months, for as long as remission is not achieved. Structural damage should be assessed by radiographs of hands and feet every 6–12 months during the first few years. Functional assessment can be used to complement this monitoring.

The recommendations note that the great variety of available therapies, together with the heterogeneity of this patient group, means that management according to fixed protocols will become more difficult. Treatment should be tailored to the individual needs of every patient.

In terms of future progress, the committee noted that there is a need to develop new tools for the accurate and early diagnosis of rheumatoid arthritis and the assessment of prognosis. Such tools might include imaging and serology measures and predictive algorithms.

BSR guidelines

The British Society for Rheumatology and the British Health Professionals in Rheumatology have produced a guideline for the management of rheumatoid arthritis in the first 2 years (Luqmani et al. 2006). It aims to give practical advice on how best to use the currently available services and outlines the evidence in support of the effectiveness of interventions for rheumatoid arthritis. It emphasises a team approach in management, and covers control of symptoms and signs; self-management by patients; methods for improving physical functioning, such as physiotherapy and occupational therapy; psychosocial function; and screening monitoring. It does not aim to give detailed recommendations about the use of DMARDs or biologic therapies because these matters are covered in other guidelines.

An algorithm summarising the BRS recommendations for the management of early rheumatoid arthritis is given in Figure 7.1.

NICE guidance

The National Institute of Health and Clinical Excellence (NICE) guidance on rheumatoid arthritis (NICE 2009) is based on systematic reviews of the best available evidence and, when minimal or no evidence is found, on the opinion of the guideline development group as to what constitutes good practice. It does not look specifically at early rheumatoid arthritis in the main body of the text, but the on-line Appendix C to the full version of the guideline [National Institute for Clinical Excellence (NICE) and National Collaborating Centre for Chronic Conditions 2009] does provide a cost–utility analysis of DMARDs in early disease.

In recent-onset disease, the NICE guidance recommends that C-reactive protein and key components of activity disease, such as DAS28, are measured monthly until disease is controlled to an agreed level. For treatment of newly diagnosed disease, NICE recommends:

- A combination of conventional DMARDs and biologic agents (including methotrexate plus at least one other DMARD, and short-term glucocorticoids) should be instituted as soon as possible.
- Where combination therapy is not appropriate, DMARD monotherapy should be used, concentrating more on fast escalation until there is sustained and satisfactory disease control than on the choice of DMARD.
- When sustained and satisfactory disease control has been achieved, there should be cautious dose-reduction to a level that continues to maintain control.

Finally, as a key priority, NICE recommends that all patients with rheumatoid arthritis should have access to a named member of the multidisciplinary team who coordinates their care.

Algorithm for the management of RA in the first 2 years.

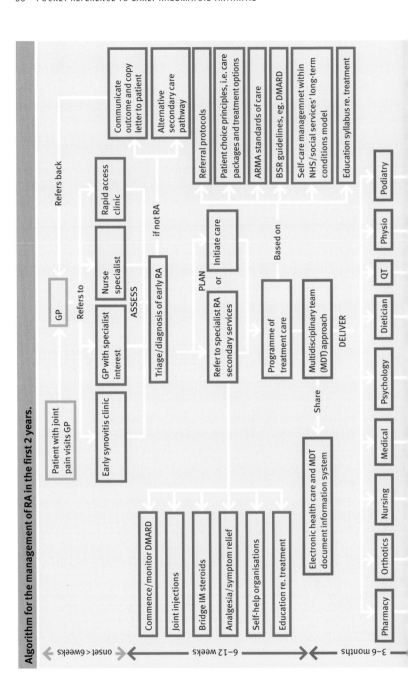

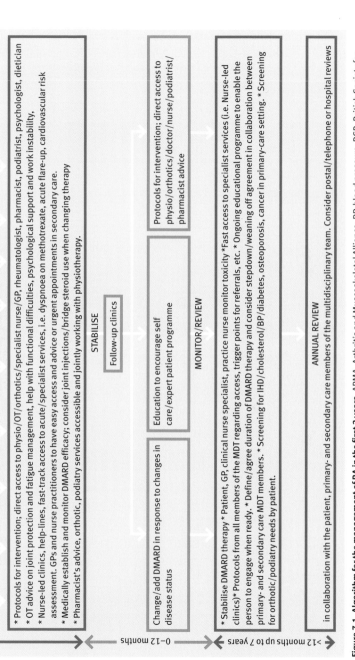

Figure 7.1. Algorithm for the management of RA in the first 2 years. ARMA, Arthritis and Musculoskeletal Alliance; BP, blood pressure; BSR, British Society for Rheumatology; DMARD, disease-modifying antirheumatic drug; GP, general practitioner; IHD, ischaemic heart disease; IM, intramuscular; OT, occupational therapy; RA, rheumatoid arthritis. Reproduced with permission from Luqmani et al. 2006.

Ikeda I, Cox S, Emery P. Aspects of early arthritis. Biological therapy in early arthritis: overtreatment or the way to go? Arthritis Res Ther 2007;9:211–217.

Jacobi CE, Mol GD, Boshuizen HC, et al. Impact of socioeconomic status on the course of rheumatoid arthritis and on related use of health care services. Arthritis Rheum 2003;49:567–573.

Jansen LM, van der Horst-Bruinsma IE, van Schaardenburg D, et al. Predictors of radiographic joint damage in patients with early rheumatoid arthritis. Ann Rheum Dis 2001;60:924–927.

John S, Myerscough A, Marlow A, et al. Linkage of cytokine genes to rheumatoid arthritis. Evidence of genetic homogeneity. Ann Rheum Dis 1998;57:361–365.

Kalla AA, Tikly M. Rheumatoid arthritis in the developing world. Best Pract Res Clin Rheumatol 2003;17:863–875.

Kane D, Balint PV, Sturrock RD. Ultrasonography is superior to clinical examination in the detection and localization of knee joint effusion in rheumatoid arthritis. J Rheumatol 2003;30:966–971.

Kavanaugh A, Rosengren S, Lee SJ, et al. Assessment of rituximab's immunomodulatory synovial effects (ARISE trial). 1: clinical and synovial biomarker results. Ann Rheum Dis 2008;67:402–408.

Kazis LE, Callahan LF, Meenan RF, et al. Health status reports in the care of patients with rheumatoid arthritis. J Clin Epidemiol 1990;43:1243–1253.

Keystone E, Emery P, Peterfy CG, et al. Rituximab inhibits structural joint damage in patients with rheumatoid arthritis with an inadequate response to tumour necrosis factor inhibitor therapies. Ann Rheum Dis 2009;68:216–221.

King YE, Watson KD, Symmons DP, et al. Pregnancy outcome in women exposed to anti-TNF agents: an update from the British Society for Rheumatology Biologics Register (BSRBR). Abstract 1011 presented at American College of Rheumatology 2008 Annual Scientific Meeting, San Francisco, October 2008. [http://acr.confex.com/acr/2008/webprogram/Paper3141.html; accessed 30 October 2009]

Kirwan J. The effect of glucocorticoids on joint destruction in rheumatoid arthritis. The Arthritis and Rheumatism Council Low-Dose Glucocorticoid Study Group. N Engl J Med 1995;333:142–146.

Klareskog L, Stolt P, Lundberg K, et al. A new model for an etiology of rheumatoid arthritis: smoking may trigger HLA–DR (shared epitope)–restricted immune reactions to autoantigens modified by citrullination. Arthritis Rheum 2006;54:38–46.

Klaukka T, Kaarela K. Methotrexate is the leading DMARD in Finland. Ann Rheum Dis 2003;62:494–496.

Kremer JM, Dougados M, Emery P, et al. Treatment of rheumatoid arthritis with the selective costimulation modulator abatacept: twelve-month results of a phase iib, double-blind, randomized, placebo-controlled trial. Arthritis Rheum 2005;52:2263–2271. Erratum in: Arthritis Rheum 2005;52:3321.

Landewe RB, Boers M, Verhoeven AC, et al. COBRA combination therapy in patients with early rheumatoid arthritis: long-term structural benefits of a brief intervention. Arthritis Rheum 2002;46:347–356.

Larsen A, Dale K, Eek M. Radiographic evaluation of rheumatoid arthritis and related conditions by standard reference films. Acta Radiol Diagn (Stockh) 1977;18:481–491.

Lee HS, Irigoyen P, Kern M, et al. Interaction between smoking, the shared epitope, and anti-cyclic citrullinated peptide: a mixed picture in three large North American rheumatoid arthritis cohorts. Arthritis Rheum 2007;56: 1745–1753.

Leeb BF, Haindl PM, Maktari A, et al. Disease activity score-28 values differ considerably depending on patient's pain perception and sex. J Rheumatol 2007;34:2382–2387.

Leombruno JP, Einarson TR, Keystone EC. The safety of anti-tumour necrosis factor treatments in rheumatoid arthritis: meta and exposure-adjusted pooled analyses of serious adverse events.Ann Rheum Dis 2009;68:1136–1145.

Listing J, Strangfeld A, Kekow J, et al. Does tumor necrosis factor alpha inhibition promote or prevent heart failure in patients with rheumatoid arthritis? Arthritis Rheum 2008;58:667–677.

Lozeron P, Denier C, Lacroix C, et al. Long-term course of demyelinating neuropathies occurring during tumor necrosis factor-alpha-blocker therapy. Arch Neurol 2009;66:490–497.

Luqmani R, Hennell S, Estrach C, et al.; on behalf of the British Society for Rheumatology and British Health Professionals in Rheumatology Standards, Guidelines and Audit Working Group. British Society for Rheumatology and British Health Professionals in Rheumatology guideline for the management of rheumatoid arthritis (the first 2 years). Rheumatology (Oxford) 2006;45:1167–1169. [http://rheumatology.oxfordjournals.org/cgi/reprint/kel215b?ijkey=0kjei4dN1B7Gmgz&keytype=ref]

Machold KP, Stamm TA, Nell VP, et al. Very recent onset rheumatoid arthritis: clinical and serological patient characteristics associated with radiographic progression over the first years of disease. Rheumatology (Oxford) 2007;46:342–349.

Maiden N, Capell HA, Madhok R, et al. Does social disadvantage contribute to the excess mortality in rheumatoid arthritis patients? Ann Rheum Dis 1999;58:525–529.

Maini RN, Taylor PC, Szechinski J, et al. Double-blind randomized controlled clinical trial of the interleukin-6 receptor antagonist, tocilizumab, in European patients with rheumatoid arthritis who had an incomplete response to methotrexate. Arthritis Rheum 2006;54:2817–2829.

Marra CA, Lynd LD, Esdaile JM, et al. The impact of low family income on self-reported health outcomes in patients with rheumatoid arthritis within a publicly funded health-care environment. Rheumatology (Oxford) 2004;43:1390–1397.

McQueen FM, Ostergaard M. Established rheumatoid arthritis: new imaging modalities. Best Pract Res Clin Rheumatol 2007;21:841–856.

McQueen FM, Benton N, Perry D, et al. Bone edema scored on magnetic resonance imaging scans of the dominant carpus at presentation predicts radiographic joint damage of the hands and feet six years later in patients with rheumatoid arthritis. Arthritis Rheum 2003;48:1814–1827.

Möttönen T, Hannonen P, Korpela M, et al. Delay to institution of therapy and induction of remission using single-drug or combination-disease-modifying antirheumatic drug therapy in early rheumatoid arthritis. Arthritis Rheum 2002;46:894–898.

Nam J, Combe B, Emery P. Early arthritis: diagnosis and management. EULAR On-line Course on Rheumatic Diseases, Module no. 13. [http://www.eular.org/index.cfm?framePage=/edu_online_course.cfm; accessed 18 July 2009]

National Audit Office. Services for people with rheumatoid arthritis. Report by the Comptroller and Auditor General HC 823 Session 2008–2009, 15 July 2009. London: The Stationery Office, 2009. [http://www.nao.org.uk/idoc.ashx?docId=3884f599-9c81-4976-aa4b-4ebebbf2dba3&version=-1; accessed 17 August 2009]

National Institute for Clinical Excellence (NICE). Rituximab for the treatment of rheumatoid arthritis. NICE technology appraisal guidance 126. London: NICE, 2007. [http://www.nice.org.uk/nicemedia/pdf/TA126guidance.pdf; accessed 9 September 2009]

National Institute for Clinical Excellence (NICE). Abatacept for the treatment of rheumatoid arthritis. NICE technology appraisal guidance 141. London: NICE, 2008. [http://www.nice.org.uk/nicemedia/pdf/TA126guidance.pdf; accessed 9 September 2009]

National Institute for Clinical Excellence (NICE). Rheumatoid arthritis. The management of rheumatoid arthritis in adults. NICE Clinical guideline 79. London: NICE, 2009.

National Institute for Clinical Excellence (NICE) and National Collaborating Centre for Chronic Conditions. Rheumatoid arthritis: national clinical guideline for management and treatment in adults. London: Royal College of Physicians, 2009. [http://www.nice.org.uk/nicemedia/pdf/CG79FullGuideline.pdf; accessed 18 July 2009; http://www.rcplondon.ac.uk/pubs/contents/6e965217-59a4-4848-8eb3-db8fc6bde333.pdf; accessed 30 July 2009]

Nasir A, Greenberg JD. TNF antagonist safety in rheumatoid arthritis: updated evidence from observational registries. Bull NYU Hosp Jt Dis 2007;65:178–181.

Nell VP, Machold KP, Eberl G, et al. Benefit of very early referral and very early therapy with disease-modifying anti-rheumatic drugs in patients with early rheumatoid arthritis. Rheum catology 2004;43:906–914.

Nishimoto N, Hashimoto J, Miyasaka N, et al. Study of active controlled monotherapy used for rheumatoid arthritis, an IL-6 inhibitor (SAMURAI): evidence of clinical and radiographic benefit from an X ray reader-blinded randomised controlled trial of tocilizumab. Ann Rheum Dis 2007;66:1162-1167.

Odegård S, Finset A, Mowinckel P, et al. Pain and psychological health status over a 10-year period in patients with recent onset rheumatoid arthritis. Ann Rheum Dis 2007;66:1195–1201.

Ohsugi Y, Kishimoto T. The recombinant humanized anti-IL-6 receptor antibody tocilizumab, an innovative drug for the treatment of rheumatoid arthritis. Expert Opin Biol Ther 2008;8:669–681.

Olsen NJ, Stein CM. New drugs for rheumatoid arthritis. N Engl J Med 2004;350:2167–2179.

Pinals RS, Masi AT, Larsen RA. Preliminary criteria for clinical remission in rheumatoid arthritis. Arthritis Rheum 1981;24:1308–1315.

Pincus T, Callahan LF. Taking mortality in rheumatoid arthritis seriously—predictive markers, socioeconomic status and comorbidity. J Rheumatol 1986;13:841–845.

Pincus T, Brooks RH, Callahan LF. Prediction of long-term mortality in patients with rheumatoid arthritis according to simple questionnaire and joint count measures. Ann Intern Med 1994;120:26–34.

Pincus T, O'Dell JR, Kremer JM. Combination therapy with multiple disease-modifying antirheumatic drugs in rheumatoid arthritis: a preventive strategy. Ann Intern Med 1999;131:768–774.

Pratt AG, Isaacs JD, Mattey DL. Current concepts in the pathogenesis of early rheumatoid arthritis. Best Pract Res Clin Rheumatol 2009;23:37–48.

Prevoo ML, van Gestel AM, van 't Hof MA, et al. Remission in a prospective study of patients with rheumatoid arthritis. American Rheumatism Association preliminary remission criteria in relation to the disease activity score. Br J Rheumatol 1996;35:1101–1105.

Quinn MA, Green MJ, Marzo-Ortega H, et al. Prognostic factors in a large cohort of patients with early undifferentiated inflammatory arthritis after application of a structured management protocol. Arthritis Rheum 2003;48:3039–3045.

Quinn MA, Conaghan PG, O'Connor PJ, et al. Very early treatment with infliximab in addition to methotrexate in early, poor-prognosis rheumatoid arthritis reduces magnetic resonance imaging evidence of synovitis and damage, with sustained benefit after infliximab withdrawal: results from a twelve-month randomized, double-blind, placebo-controlled trial. Arthritis Rheum 2005;52:27–35.

Rindfleisch JA, Muller D. Diagnosis and management of rheumatoid arthritis. Am Fam Physician 2005;72:1037–1047.

Rostom A, Dubé C, Jolicoeur E, et al. Gastro-duodenal ulcers associated with the use of non-steroidal anti-inflammatory drugs: a systematic review of preventive pharmacological interventions. Ottawa: Canadian Coordinating Office for Health Technology Assessment; 2003: Technology report No 38.

Saag KG, Teng GG, Patkar NM, et al. American College of Rheumatology 2008 recommendations for the use of nonbiologic and biologic disease-modifying antirheumatic drugs in rheumatoid arthritis. Arthritis Rheum 2008;49:762–784.

Scottish Intercollegiate Guidelines Network. Management of early rheumatoid arthritis. Guideline no. 48. Edinburgh: Scottish Intercollegiate Guidelines Network, 2000. [http://www.sign.ac.uk/pdf/sign48.pdf; accessed 26 June 2009]

Setoguchi S. Solomon DH, Weinblatt ME, et al. Tumor necrosis factor α antagonist use and cancer in patients with rheumatoid arthritis. Arthritis Rheum 2006;54:2757–2764.

Sharp JT, Lidsky MD, Collins LC, et al. Methods of scoring the progression of radiologic changes in rheumatoid arthritis. Arthritis Rheum 1971;14:706–720.

Silman AJ. The changing face of rheumatoid arthritis: why the decline in incidence? Arthritis Rheum 2002;26:579–581.

Singh JA, Christensen R, Wells GA, et al. Biologics for rheumatoid arthritis: an overview of Cochrane reviews. Cochrane Database of Systematic Reviews 2009;4:CD007848. [DOI: 10.1002/14651858.CD007848.pub2]

Smolen JS, Han C, Bala M, et al. Evidence of radiographic benefit of treatment with infliximab plus methotrexate in rheumatoid arthritis patients who had no clinical improvement: a detailed subanalysis of data from the anti-tumor necrosis factor trial in rheumatoid arthritis with concomitant therapy study. Arthritis Rheum 2005;52:1020–1030.

Smolen JS, Beaulieu A, Rubbert-Roth A, et al. Effect of interleukin-6 receptor inhibition with tocilizumab in patients with rheumatoid arthritis (OPTION study): a double-blind, placebo-controlled,randomised trial. Lancet 2008;371:987–997.

Smolen JS, Steiner G. Therapeutic strategies for rheumatoid arthritis. Nat Rev Drug Discov 2003;2:473–488.

Sokka T. Radiographic scoring in rheumatoid arthritis: a short introduction to the methods. Bull NYU Hosp Jt Dis 2008;66:166–168.

Sokka TM, Kautiainen HJ, Hannonen PJ. A retrospective study of treating RA patients with various combinations of slow-acting antirheumatic drugs in a county hospital. Scand J Rheumatol 1997;26:440–443.

Sommer OJ, Kladosek A, Weiler V, et al. Rheumatoid arthritis: a practical guide to state-of-the-art imaging, image interpretation, and clinical implications. RadioGraphics 2005;25:381–398.

St Clair EW, van der Heijde DM, Smolen JS, et al. Combination of infliximab and methotrexate therapy for early rheumatoid arthritis: a randomized, controlled trial. Arthritis Rheum 2004;50:3432–3443.

Stone M, Bergin D, Whelan B, et al. Power Doppler ultrasound assessment of rheumatoid hand synovitis. J Rheumatol 2001;28:1979–1982.

Strand V, Sokolove J. Randomized controlled trial design in rheumatoid arthritis: the past decade. Arthritis Res Ther 2009, 11:205–215.

Strand V, Mease P, Burmester GR, et al. Rapid and sustained improvements in health-related quality of life, fatigue, and other patient-reported outcomes in rheumatoid arthritis patients treated with certolizumab pegol plus methotrexate over 1 year: results from the RAPID 1 randomized controlled trial. Arthritis Res Ther. 2009 Nov 12;11(6):R170. [Epub ahead of print]

Stübgen JP. Tumor necrosis factor-alpha antagonists and neuropathy. Muscle Nerv 2008;37:281–292.

Sugimoto H, Takeda A, Hyodoh K. Early-stage rheumatoid arthritis: prospective study of the effectiveness of MR imaging for diagnosis. Radiology 2000;216:569–575.

Summary of Product Characteristics for Cimzia (certolizumab). [http://www.emea.europa.eu/humandocs/PDFs/EPAR/cimzia/emea-combined-h1037en.pdf]

Summary of Product Characteristics for Embrel (etanercept). [http://www.emea.europa.eu/humandocs/PDFs/EPAR/Enbrel/emea-combined-h262en.pdf]

Summary of Product Characteristics for Humira (abatacept). [http://www.emea.europa.eu/humandocs/PDFs/EPAR/humira/emea-combined-h481en.pdf]

Summary of Product Characteristics for MabThera (rituximab). [http://www.emea.europa.eu/humandocs/PDFs/EPAR/Mabthera/emea-combined-h165en.pdf

Summary of Product Characteristics for Orencia (abatacept). [http://www.emea.europa.eu/humandocs/PDFs/EPAR/orencia/emea-combined-h701en.pdf]

Summary of Product Characteristics for Remicade (infliximab). [http://www.emea.europa.eu/humandocs/PDFs/EPAR/Remicade/emea-combined-h240en.pdf]

Summary of Product Characteristics for RoActemra (tocilizumab). [http://www.emea.europa.eu/humandocs/PDFs/EPAR/RoActemra/H-955-PI-en.pdf]

Suresh E. Diagnosis of early rheumatoid arthritis: what the non-specialist needs to know. J R Soc Med 2004;97:421–424.

Tak P, Bresnihan B. The pathogenesis and prevention of joint damage in rheumatoid arthritis. Advances from synovial biopsy and tissue analysis. Arthritis Rheum 2000;43:2619–2633.

van der Heijde D. How to read radiographs according to the Sharp/van der Heijde method. J Rheumatol 1999;26:743–745.

van der Heijde DM. Radiographic imaging: the 'gold standard' for assessment of disease progression in rheumatoid arthritis. Rheumatology (Oxford) 2000;39 (Suppl. 1):9–16.

van der Heijde D, Boers M, Lassere M. Methodological issues in radiographic scoring methods in rheumatoid arthritis. J Rheumatol 1999;26:726–730.

van der Helm-van Mil AH, Huizinga TW, de Vries RR, et al. Emerging patterns of risk factor make-up enable subclassification of rheumatoid arthritis. Arthritis Rheum 2007a;56:1728–1735.

van der Helm-van Mil AH, le Cessie S, van Dongen H, et al. A prediction rule for disease outcome in patients with recent-onset undifferentiated arthritis: how to guide individual treatment decisions. Arthritis Rheum 2007b;56:433–440.

van der Horst-Bruinsma IE, Speyer I, Visser H, et al. Diagnosis and course of early onset arthritis: results of a special early arthritis clinic compared to routine patient care. Br J Rheumatol 1998;37:1084–1088.

van Dongen H, van Aken J, Lard LR, et al. Efficacy of methotrexate treatment in patients with probable rheumatoid arthritis: a double-blind, randomized, placebo-controlled trial. Arthritis Rheum 2007;56:1424–1432.

van Everdingen AA, Jacobs JW, Siewertsz van Reesema DR, et al. Low-dose prednisone therapy for patients with early active rheumatoid arthritis: clinical efficacy, disease-modifying properties, and side effects: a randomized, double-blind, placebo-controlled clinical trial. Ann Intern Med 2002;136:1–12.

van Gestel AM, Prevoo ML, van 't Hof MA, et al. Development and validation of the European League Against Rheumatism response criteria for rheumatoid arthritis. Comparison with the preliminary American College of Rheumatology and the World Health Organization/ International League Against Rheumatism Criteria. Arthritis Rheum 1996;39:34–40.

van Riel PLCM, Schumacher HR. How does one assess early rheumatoid arthritis in daily clinical practice? Best Pract Res Clin Rheumatol 2001;15:67–76.

Verpoort KN, van Dongen H, Allaart CF, et al. Undifferentiated arthritis: disease course assessed in several inception cohorts. Clin Exp Rheumatol 2004;22 (Suppl. 35):S12–S17.

Visser H, le Cessie S, Vos K, et al. How to diagnose rheumatoid arthritis early: a prediction model for persistent (erosive) arthritis. Arthritis Rheum 2002;46:357–365.

Vos K, Thurlings RM, Wijbrandts CA, et al. Early effects of rituximab on the synovial cell infiltrate in patients with rheumatoid arthritis. Arthritis Rheum 2007;56:772–778.

Wakefield RJ, Gibbon WW, Conaghan PG, et al. The value of sonography in the detection of bone erosions in patients with rheumatoid arthritis: a comparison with conventional radiography. Arthritis Rheum 2000;43:2762–2770.

Wamser G, Bohndorf K, Vollert K, et al. Power Doppler sonography with and without echo-enhancing contrast agent and contrast-enhanced MRI for the evaluation of rheumatoid arthritis of the shoulder joint: differentiation between synovitis and joint effusion. Skeletal Radiol 2003;32:351–359.

Weinblatt ME. Rheumatoid arthritis: more aggressive approach improves outlook. Cleve Clin J Med 2004;71:409–413.

Weinblatt M, Combe B, Covucci A, et al. Safety of the selective costimulation modulator abatacept in rheumatoid arthritis patients receiving background biologic and nonbiologic disease-modifying antirheumatic drugs: a one-year randomized, placebo-controlled study. Arthritis Rheum 2006;54:2807–2816.

Weusten BL, Jacobs J, Bijlsma J. Corticosteroid pulse therapy in active RA. Semin Arthritis Rheum 1993;23:183–192.

Weyand CM, Hicok KC, Conn DL, et al. The influence of HLA-DRB1 genes on disease severity in rheumatoid arthritis. Ann Intern Med 1992;15;117:801–806.

Wienecke T, Gotzsche PC. Paracetamol versus nonsteroidal anti-inflammatory drugs for rheumatoid arthritis. Cochrane Database Syst Rev 2004:CD003789.

Williams EL, Gadola S, Edwards CJ. Anti-TNF-induced lupus. Rheumatology 2009;48:716–720.

Wolfe F, Hawley DJ. Remission in rheumatoid arthritis. J Rheumatol 1985;12:245–252.

Wolfe F, Michaud K. Biologic treatment of rheumatoid arthritis and the risk of malignancy analyses from a large US observational study. Arthritis Rheum 2007;56:2886–2895.

Yelin E, Wanke LA. An assessment of the annual and long-term direct costs of rheumatoid arthritis: the impact of poor function and functional decline. Arthritis Rheum 1999;42:1209–1218.